"I have always thought that I was very big boned and was made just right to be an athlete. I excepted my size because that was how athletes were, right? After having my 4 babies things were not the same, I didn't feel like I looked like that athlete anymore. Even with rigorous training, lifting weights and running, I couldn't get back to my before baby weight. I decided to get on Janette Hansen's "Taming the Monster Within" program and when I committed to her plan things began to change. I was not going to vary, as I had decided I was going to do this exactly as Janette laid out in her program. It was a surprise that I had to limit my fruit intake because that was what I ate all day and thought it was the healthiest thing for me. I found out I was addicted to the sugar in the fruit.

"When the weight started coming off it never really stopped. I had a few plateaus but really the progress was steady. I have lost 80 pounds in about 8 months. Sometimes were hard, but it has gotten easy as this is now my lifestyle. I am at maintenance and I am enjoying this new me. I have confidence to be able to meet new people and feel proud about how I look. I have taught my family about the dangers of sugar. My children have made changes in their life as well which is so important for their health and wellbeing in their future. I have really appreciated Janette's counseling, she gave me the information I needed to be successful. This plan works! "

Dodie Beavin, Independence, Idaho

"I've lost 65 pounds so far following Janette's plan. I feel confident knowing her plan is backed by science and is nutritionally sound. For the first time in my adult life I'm confident and hopeful for the future. I feel like this is has been an answer to prayer. I've never lost this much weight before, and I'm still going!"

Tenise Wertman, Rexburg, Idaho

"The weight has crept up on me through the years. I used to be a size 10 and because I am tall that was a great size for me. Without realizing it I had become addicted to sugar and gained weight. With my job and the stress of life I felt helpless to do anything about it. I would try low carb diets but even with my resolve they just didn't work. The "Taming the Monster Within" program gave me an understanding of what was going on and what the real problem was. I have lost 60 pounds and feel so much better with so much more energy. I am not worried about gaining it back as I have a new lifestyle that is awesome. I know the way I will eat for the rest of my life and it is liberating. I plan for my indulgences but I can stop and get back on track right away so it's all good. I do not feel that I have to deprive myself, it's just delayed gratification."

Victoria Grant, Paterson, California

"I used to hate getting ready to go out to dinner and things like that because I didn't like how I looked and I was tired all the time but that is changing. It's been hard and I really have to pay attention to what I'm eating but it is getting easier. I really do feel better both physically and mentally. I have lost 25 pounds and plan on continuing until I reach goal. Then I will go into the maintenance portion of the program. I plan on this being my new lifestyle for life. The rewards are too good to ever go back."

Natalee Riley, Burton, Idaho

"After being a police officer for Dade County, Florida for many years, I was excited about retirement. Being an officer kept me in shape, but as a retiree, well, that has its own challenges. With civilian life it's just too easy to not do those rigorous workouts anymore. Also my blood tests that came back from my yearly exams were nothing to be happy with. I gained over 80 pounds and was at a loss as to how I should lose it. I tried doing what I thought was the correct thing nutritionally and still kept gaining weight. When Janette started to counsel me she said "You have to do exactly what I tell you, no mistakes." I was so sick of the weight that I was ready for that. When I agreed, there was no turning back. I made the changes necessary, and stuck to it no matter what. I even gave away my clothes that had become too big to people who could use them. It all worked and in a matter of months I lost 87 pounds. If I start to gain I get right back to the basics. I feel so good and at my yearly exams the doctors are proud of me. I am proud of me too!"

Eve Mucci, Charlotte, North Carolina.

Taming the Monster Within

A guide to overcoming sugar addiction, losing weight, keeping it off, and not being afraid of the sugar "Monster" ever again

by

Janette Hansen

New Day Wellness Publications
4030 S 5500 W
Rexburg, Idaho 83440
www.TamingtheMonsterWithin.com

New Day Wellness Publications is a division of New Day Wellness LLC

Cover design by Amanda Price
Author photo by Chris Godfrey

Dedication

This book is for my husband, Brent, and my children and their spouses, who are also my children but just from another mother: Josh & Rachelle, Ben & JaNell, Samantha & Daimon, Amanda & Blake, Jessica & Kyle, Heather & Matt, and Whitney & Cameron; and also our grandchildren.

Table of Contents

Disclaimer

Before you begin any program that will affect your health in any way you should talk to your licensed health care provider. *"Taming the Monster Within"* is not intended as a substitute for the advice and/or medical care of the reader's physician. Any lifestyle regime should be under the direct supervision of the reader's physician. Nothing in this book is intended to diagnose, treat, cure, or prevent disease. The information in this book is for educational purposes only and is not intended to replace or adjust any information contained on or in any product label or packaging. Janette Hansen is a nutritician and does not claim to be an expert in any illness, disease, or treatment. In this book she is merely sharing one of her interests.

Acknowledgements

This book would never have been written if it were not for my clients who inspire and teach me. As they strive for something better, I keep striving for more knowledge. My family and friends have been so encouraging that it actually made me think I could do this. My sisters, Chris and Vicky, never doubted me and helped with their great thoughts and editing. I want to thank Amanda Price for her graphic artist talents which brought the concept of this book to life with the cover image. Gail Taylor was able to whip this book into shape by her final editing. Jeff Thomason helped me format and prepare this book for publishing. My sincere gratitude to them all. My Heavenly Father kept putting the ideas out there in front of me at a pace I could keep up with. He leads me along and I have faith in his help. I could not do it without him.

Introduction

I had been a student of nutrition long before I got my degree and long before I started counseling people on their diets. Years ago I was a dialysis technician when the dialysis machine looked like a big washing machine. The procedure of cleaning a persons' blood through dialysis was relatively new.

I watched as people's health declined because nutrients were actually washed out of the blood along with the accumulated toxins. Even then I could see the importance of proper nutrition. It was an amazing procedure for the time, and even with its shortcomings, dialysis prolonged many lives.

Things have come a long way in medical science and nutritional therapies. My text books in college were far behind what was then validated research and are now accepted as truth.

I have watched as nutritional science has stumbled along, first teaching one thing and then another, dragging us along with it. It has been my pleasure to see teachings about nutrition become more enlightened.

After college, I continued to receive further training in nutritional therapies from Sanoviv Medical Center, Boise State University, and London Live Blood. I am trained and certified with Darkfield Microscopy and work under the direction of the attending physician at a several local clinics. This gives me the opportunity to see how people's diets effect their health in a very direct way.

I have been a nutritional counselor for seventeen years, helping people gain health through their diet and lifestyle. Having spent most of that time teaching about weight loss, I have watched my clients be successful in losing weight, even large amounts, and keeping their weight off when they utilize the techniques I have taught them. Usually, I see people when they have tried everything else to lose weight and get their lives in balance and nothing has had lasting effects. The first thing they learn is that being over-weight is not about a lack of character. They learn about the sinister nature of the modern diet and how they can be in control, rather than out of control.

For years I was a ski instructor, teaching the children from the local schools, until one day, after a long day of teaching beginners, I went for one last run from the top just for fun. It wasn't a very spectacular fall, but it was devastating. I had blown out my knee. The doctor did a total knee reconstruction, leaving me with significant pain during any kind of impact exercise. This was the beginning of a new exercise career for me. Water aerobics gave me the chance to get a great work out without the pain that high impact exercise brought. As I progressed I found out that exercise in the water gave the perfect opportunity for an all-over body building experience with a great cardio session as well. I have designed a program that utilizes that aspect. For over eleven years I have taught this program to the students who have attended my water aerobics class at Ricks College, then the local sports club, and now at the recreational pool in town. Exercise is such an essential part of good health and I have seen this first hand.

It is so fun and gratifying for me to see people change their lives and be happy and proud of their accomplishments. Losing weight, getting in shape, and controlling addictions is a powerful life changer for the better. I truly believe when people are properly taught correct information, they will come to know and act upon that truth for themselves. Their success is what inspires me and keeps me on the learning path.

I am just the teacher who will always be a student.

Recognizing the "Monster Within"

You may ask "What's wrong with me?"...Nothing...except you LOVE Donuts!!! I mean you REALLY LOVE donuts!!!

Have you ever lost weight, maybe even a lot of weight and felt pretty great about things? Maybe you bought the program off the TV, or you went to a counselor, maybe you bought a book and studied information about weight loss, then added a regular exercise regime! Yeah, you look pretty darn good.

Well, Emily, a client of mine, had done just that. She had lost 24 pounds. One night she invited the family over for a fun movie evening, and she made them a great big bowl of caramel popcorn. It was delicious (she's a great cook), and eating in front of everyone made her especially happy because she was thin so she felt she could. The freedom was exhilarating! Her guests went home and while she was cleaning up she started snacking on the leftover popcorn, eating until her stomach hurt, but she still kept eating. She started to think, "What's going on here, why can't I stop? What's wrong with me? "

This was wrong on every level but that sweet caramel popcorn was so amazing, she thought she might as well finish it. Actually, at this point her ability to stop was not really there. She began to be disappointed in herself, almost to self-loathing. Emily looked at herself in the mirror and was disgusted, thinking what a weak person she was.

STOP RIGHT THERE!

I want to tell you that the monstrous behavior she just exhibited was not her fault. It has nothing, I repeat, nothing to do with character.

People are trying to overcome not only an insulin reaction which lowers blood sugar and causes hunger but also what is now known as a real life, verifiable addiction. One that is eight times more addictive than cocaine, four times more addictive than heroin.

You have the cards stacked so firmly against you that very few people are able to overcome the dreaded insulin reaction and sugar addiction by sheer willpower.

It is such a strong force to put a processed carbohydrate in your mouth that very nice people have been known to eat a random chocolate chip that rolled under the toe kick of the cabinet. No, you don't know how long it's been there, but does it really matter? You just wish you had spilled more the last time you made cookies. If you had been thinking ahead you probably would have.

For those of you who have a challenge with their weight and are tired of losing pounds only to gain them back, just confirming what you suspected, you are out of control, well I have help for you.

It's time to bring out the truth and let the chips fall where they may. (Did you think I meant chocolate chips?)

Let's look at how we have gotten our society into this predicament.

The History of the Monster

Sugar, derived from fruits and honey, existed from the beginning of man's history. The availability to obtain fresh fruit would have been seasonal and the surplus would likely have been dried out in the sun, for example, changing grapes into raisins and plums into prunes. Other common fruits in ancient times were figs, pears, dates, cherries and peaches.

But first you had to have access to those foods. You couldn't just pop into the grocery store and pick whatever your heart desired. The point is that availability was limited for most so the damage that comes from prolonged high blood sugar was very limited as well.

Type 1 Diabetes was written about in ancient history texts. It was called the sweet urine disease, and the cause of it was not known. Type 1 Diabetes was most likely a death sentence in ancient days.

The ancient Egyptians used honey as a sweetener, as a gift to their gods and even as an ingredient in embalming fluid. Hippocrates used it as a base for most of his formulations and medicines.

Reading about the use of honey in historical writings places it firmly in human consumption but the idea that it was used as commonly as sugar is today is not probable. The probable thing is that it was used sparingly and with purpose. After all, when you have to deal with beehives and busy bees, you will value what you get and not waste it. If you could not or would not have the access to beehives, buying honey would have been very expensive.

For the purpose of this book, which is being able to live a healthy lifestyle and get a handle on one's sugar addiction, honey is sugar. However, keeping in mind that our ancestors had modest sweet intake and that Dr. Keith Kantor, PHD, a nutritionist has been quoted saying that "honey consists of 30% glucose and less than 40% fructose, as well as 20 other sugars in the mix, many of which are much more complex, and dextrin, a type of starchy fiber that means your body expends more energy to break it all down to glucose. Therefore, you end up accumulating fewer calories from it"(1). Honey would therefore not be considered malicious.

So when did man actually start eating processed sugar? It's thought that the people of New Guinea were probably the first to domesticate sugarcane. From there it spread to India. "In 510 BC Emperor Darius, of what was then Persia, invaded India where he found "the reed which gives honey without the bees"(2).

Sugar's cultivation spread rapidly when the Arabs learned the secret from the Persians. As the Arabs extended their sphere of influence in the world, their knowledge of sugar spread. There are records of sugar cane fields in Spain in 1444. Historical texts tell us that in 1788 the French were consuming 2.2 pounds of sugar per head per year. This sugar was predominately from sugar cane.

Sugar beets were just starting to make an appearance, and by the 1840's France had fifty-eight sugar-beet factories. Europe was on its way to being self-sufficient.

Britain was still relying on cane sugar from the colonies in the West Indies until the 20th century. In 1874, the British Prime Minister William Ewart Gladstone, abolished the sugar tax which brought down its price so it became affordable to the majority of the population (3). From that time sugar consumption has increased yearly worldwide, so much so that in the United States it's estimated at 150 to 170 pounds per person in the year 2014 (4).

I bring you this bit of history for one reason, to make the point that billions of the inhabitants of this earth, the majority of all mankind that has ever lived, did not have processed sugars. Practically speaking, it did not come into common use until the 1700's and that's being generous. Most people could not afford the "sweet salt" as it was called by the Crusaders in the 12th century (ibid). Not until the 18th and 19th centuries has it become cheap enough for common human consumption.

So how is it that modern man finds a way to put processed sugar into everything possible? This may seem simplistic, but, yes, you guessed it. MONEY.

Let's go back to the 1970"s when I was wearing bell bottom pants and desperately trying to straighten my curly hair!

We were loving the music of the Carpenters, Diana Ross, Chicago, the Bee Gees, K.C. and the Sunshine Band, Abba, and watching the Beatles break apart into individual artists. VCRs were introduced, which meant you could stay at home and watch the movie of your choice for the first time.

Society was completely oblivious to the fact that research was being done to heighten the addictiveness of sugar!

We were engaged in the Viet Nam War and the US Army was in a bind. The soldiers were having a hard time keeping their weight up, you see, MRE, which stands for "Meals Ready to Eat, had to have a shelf life of 3 months. That requirement was an appetite suppressant. How could you make food tasty and last in a package in scorching heat for three months?

The military found a guy that could help. His name was Howard Moskowitz and he was just graduating from Harvard with a PHD in experimental psychology. The Army recruited him to help them make MREs that would keep the soldiers eating.

The problem was that when the men went into combat, and the MRE's had lost their appeal, the soldiers lost body weight.

There was no specific science to this yet, but Moskowitz developed one. There were the issues of potent spicy foods, which would satiate the body quickly, and salt, as salt was becoming a health issue in the minds of many. But sugar, ah, that was what was keeping people coming back for more. We really didn't understand the addictive nature of sugar then, but Moskowitz was finding it out.

With the help of a colleague, Joseph Balintfy, they saw that the graphs developed in research showed an upside down U. The top of that U was where people ate the most, this was all about sugar mind you, and when the line went back down, people ate less. This was the "bliss point".

Moskowitz, along with the food industry, (who were ever seeking better profit margins) implemented the science of the "bliss point" into every packaged food you can think of, from spaghetti sauce and soft drinks to boxed cereal. Everything is engineered to be addictive and to keep us coming back for more, and more, and more, you get the idea.

It's a billion dollar industry, that's big bucks (5). We pay a pretty penny to satiate our sugar addiction and we're happy to do it. Can you tell me what's better than a Bavarian crème filled donut covered in chocolate icing washed down with creamy hot chocolate? "Hold the marshmallows, I'm dieting!"

There is science to this, and we are all the victims.

Defining the Monster

When I refer to the "Monster Within", it's really two fold. I am talking about the insulin reaction you experience when you eat refined foods (sugar, refined flours, and refined white rice) and I am also talking about the newly diagnosed condition that is so prevalent in our society, namely sugar addiction.

First we will discuss the part of this situation that is called the insulin reaction.

Insulin Reaction

We need to talk about what an insulin reaction is. When you eat a high carb food that causes your blood sugar levels to rise, your body will send out an alarm. Excessive levels of blood sugar will cause the body serious problems. The system knows that very high blood sugar can lead to damage in the tissues of the body. Too high of blood sugar can actually cause coma.

Insulin is a hormone made by the pancreas. With the production of insulin, sugar in the blood is lowered. It does this by putting the available carbs, which, after digestion, are now in the form of glucose, into the cells of the body and into the liver for future energy needs.

A sugar addict may have been eating so much sugar for so long that their body produces too much insulin and lowers the blood sugar too low. This is called hypoglycemia. Symptoms of hypoglycemia may include fatigue, pale skin, shakiness, anxiety, sweating, irritability, Heart palpitations and/or hunger. The hunger that occurs when a person is experiencing low blood sugar is more accurately described as cravings.

The body wants to raise its sugar levels so you will be craving the best things to do that. Examples are cookies, bread, candy, soda, chocolate, or macaroni and cheese. Say hello to the "Monster Within". Some people believe that this is a good thing because you need carbs to produce insulin. I know this because I have given lectures where people voice that opinion and they are passionate about it. I am going to type this very quietly so people who don't agree with this won't hear it. You don't have to have carbs. Nope, your body can turn protein into sugar when it is necessary. It is called gluconeogenesis. This is why you only want to eat a protein serving that is the size of the palm of your hand. That's a great indicator of what a good serving is for you. More than that may be more than your body can digest and will be turned into sugar.

I am getting ahead of myself. Just the act of eating stimulates the intestines to send the message that insulin production is needed and you will get some insulin with just protein. Insulin is what makes it possible for nutrients as well as fats to get into the cells so let's not be too hard on insulin. It is vital for life. With that said, let's see where insulin becomes the villain.

New Harvard research reported by Mark Hyman M.D. shows that where eating is involved, what stimulates the nucleus accumbens, the pleasure center of the brain, is the production of insulin.

In the study researchers took a group of obese men and gave them a milkshake that was low glycemic. The Glycemic Index measures the impact a food has on blood sugar and therefore insulin production. When a food is low glycemic that means it is slow to raise blood sugar and therefore the insulin is not spiked. When a food is high glycemic it is quick to raise the blood sugar and spikes the insulin causing an insulin reaction.

The researchers then did a brain scan to measure the reaction in the nucleus accumbens which is the pleasure center of the brain. The scan showed little stimulation.

Days later the same group was given another milkshake that matched the first one in every way: texture, protein, fat, sweetness, macronutrient content and calories, except it was high glycemic.

The participants did not know which was which as it tasted exactly the same. Unlike the first, the second milkshake lit up the nucleus accumbens like a Christmas tree. This shows two things: one, that the body reacts differently with foods that cause an insulin response and two, foods that trigger the insulin response are biologically addictive as they stimulate the nucleus accumbens, or the pleasure center of the brain.(6)

First you have the addiction to the insulin response which is simultaneous with the development of a sugar addiction. Sugar addiction is the second part of the "Monster Within" I would like to talk about.

Sugar Addiction

Sugar follows the same endorphin pathway as morphine, heroin, cocaine, tobacco, alcohol, cannabis and meth. In 2008 a study conducted by doctors NM Avena, P. Rada, and BG Hoebel figured out that the same neurochemical changes that happen in the brain in regards to drug addiction also happen with the intake of sugar. Sugar takes the same pathway as any other drug of choice and abuse. (7)

The more of the substance you intake the more it takes for you to feel the same feelings of pleasure. It's called down regulating. Because you have stimulated the dopamine receptors continually, they reduce the amount of dopamine that they produce. When you don't give the receptors the substance of choice, alcohol, tobacco, cocaine, heroin, morphine, meth, cannabis or sugar, then no dopamine is produced, and you have withdrawals.

When foods are involved, it triggers a starvation signal, and you are then in the situation where you may be trying to use cognitive inhibition to overcome a biochemical drive. In other words, you are in the bad position of attempting to use sheer will power to stop the cravings that are a physical urge. To keep steady, eating sugar may be necessary for a sugar addict just to maintain.

A medical scientist named Virginia Davis was working on a project in Houston, Texas. She was researching cancer and needed fresh human brains. She would tag along with the Houston police on their early morning rounds collecting the street alcoholics who had died that night. Using those brains she detected a chemical that is very closely related to heroin. The substance is referred to as THIQ which is short for Tetrahydroisoquinoline. (Say that fast three times!)

She mistakenly assumed that the alcoholics were taking heroin until the emergency room doctors, and the police in the area informed her that there was no way these addicts were using heroin. They could hardly afford cheap wine.

Her research showed that the sugar in the wine was releasing opioids, just like heroin does. It was leaving THIQ in the same pathway as heroin uses.(8) If a person was addicted to opioids that person would have the characteristic of being preoccupied with the desire to obtain and take the drug. They would persist in the drug seeking behavior, despite the adverse consequences from continued use and the development of withdrawal syndrome when opioid use stops(9).

Hmmmm! Think back to that person who ate the remaining bowl of caramel popcorn, to the point of discomfort and beyond. Not a pretty sight. An addiction causes a person to keep seeking and doing the behavior regardless of the consequence. Sugar creates an addiction that produces an overwhelming desire to eat more refined carbs. Eating more refined carbs creates that insulin reaction which lowers blood sugar and that alone causes hunger. Then bring in the drive to produce more endorphins in the pleasure center of the brain causing overwhelming biological cravings, and wah lah! the "Monster within"!

Deception

Recently on the front page of our local newspaper there was an article about "Exposing Sugar". (10) It was in the early 1960's that studies were being done on the relationship that sugar has to heart disease. These findings are just now coming out because the correspondence with the Harvard researchers and a sugar trade group are being uncovered.

When the sugar group heard that the research on sugar consumption showed a connection to heart disease they offered a substantial amount of money to change the verdict.

The sugar industry submitted their scientific literature that implicated fat to heart disease. They kept an eye on the content of the article produced by Harvard, which swayed public opinion and subsequent research for many years. These fraudulent articles were actually published by the New England Journal of Medicine. For decades we have been duped.

Eating Disorders

It was in 1979 that binge eating and self-induced vomiting was first given a name, "Bulimia Nervosa"(11). Anorexia existed in rare occasions in history but has become a real health hazard in the last half of the 20th century. A doctor of Evolutionary Psychiatry, Emily Deans M.D. tells us that the cases of anorexia and bulimia escalated in the 1970's and 1980's, and though some will say they peaked in that time, the national survey data suggests that bulimia especially, continues to escalate.

Most scholars will point to cultural pressures for thinness, increasing depression and obsessive compulsive behavior. These behaviors were precursors for eating disorders.

It is impossible to ignore the fact that the 1970s and 80s are when the rates of obesity in the United States began to increase at an unprecedented rate. This is also when low-fat eating began its popular progression through the mainstream.

There is a third eating disorder, binge eating disorder, where periodic food binges are not compensated by restricting or purging behavior. While many obese people eat normally, binge eaters will consume up to tens of thousands of calories in a single day. Binge eaters can consume entire bags of candy, or dinner from five or six fast food restaurants, one after the other. Again this disorder has been described for centuries, but has escalated only recently. "Binge eaters make up about 1/3 of the people who seek medical treatment for obesity."(12)

The study of these disorders is beyond the scope of this book, but to me there is a correlation to all of this. When I was a kid no one ever heard of anorexia, bulimia nervosa or binge eating. This was also at   the beginning of the "bliss point" and as an industry it was just coming into its own.

We can't blame them, it was just brilliant marketing as the dangers of sugar and sugar addiction were basically ignored by everyone. Well not everyone, but the critics were rather soft spoken.

We need to get back to the "Villain" Insulin. With so much sugar coming into our diets unwittingly, our insulin levels have risen accordingly. But many ugly things come with an increase of insulin. One of them is called insulin resistance.

Insulin Resistance

The Pancreas, weighing about 2oz, is the organ that

produces the hormone Insulin, along with glucagon and various digestive enzymes. To be more specific it is the beta cells in the Islets of Langerhans that actually produce the insulin. The islets of Langerhans make up only a small portion of the pancreas (1 to 2 percent). Get this visual in your mind. The pancreas is a small organ and only a tiny bit of that organ makes insulin.

Like all hormones, insulin is a chemical communicator. Insulin's major function is to regulate blood sugar levels. This regulation protects the brain from high sugar which can damage brain cells. Our brains are pretty important you know, in fact, it's the body's first priority. The brain relies on glucose for energy, but too much of a good thing is a bad thing.

When there is an intake of sugar, the liver takes the sugar which has been transported by the portal vein from the intestines (rich in nutrients that have been extracted from food) and produces glucose which is then escorted to the cells by insulin.

Unless you have Type 1 Diabetes, things are going pretty good. You eat proteins, fats, and unrefined carbohydrates and the body is perfectly capable of handling this. With Type 1 you will, of course, need insulin, and be under the care of your doctor, but still, with careful eating a Type 1 diabetic can live a full life.

Ok, this is where it gets tricky. When there is an intake of refined sugar like you commonly see today, soda pop, cookies, cakes, white flour anything, ketchup, candy, and the list goes on, the assault on the liver and pancreas is abnormal. Why do I call it an assault you ask? The fact is these organs were never designed for this kind of treatment. When refined foods are ingested and digested, it is like kicking the pancreas with a metal-toed boot. It is ouchy every time.

What happens to all that refined sugar? Well the liver changes it to glucose, then the insulin that the pancreas has produced can escort it to the cells for energy. Insulin is so very important in this task as it has the key necessary to open the cell door and let the glucose in. Nothing else has that ability.

When the cells become full of glucose, the liver takes in what it can store, then the rest is turned into cholesterol and triglycerides

A healthy person has a normal amount of insulin receptors in every cell. When a person eats too many high carbohydrate foods it reduces the number of insulin receptors. This happens because the cells get tired of the constant request from insulin to open the cell and take more glucose.

The cell is already full of glucose and can take no more. The cells aren't rude, just practical. Now we have what is known as insulin resistance. The definition of Insulin Resistance blames obesity as the root cause along with caloric excess, physical inactivity, genetics, and age.

Does obesity come first or does insulin resistance come first? Doesn't excessive refined sugar and flour intake cause the problem?

Remember the practical cells that reduce their number of insulin receptors? It wasn't until 1979 that the term "impaired glucose tolerance or pre-diabetes" was coined (13). The newer terminology of Type 2 Diabetes was termed between 1980 and the 1990's (14).

Let me refresh your memory, it was in the 1970's that the science of the "aha moment!" in the sugar industry was developed. That was the discovery of how much sugar it took to make a food most desirable to the point of being addictive. In the 70's Americans were consuming about 116 pounds of sugar a year per person. It has grown an estimated 19 percent by 2005(15) and then in 2017, it was about 150 to 170 pounds per person a year.

In the beginning of this trail of clues to the problem of sugar addiction and obesity, I was giving insulin and insulin reactions the brand as the "bad guy". Well, you have to blame something, and the dreaded insulin reaction seems fun to blame. I didn't want to go into the fact that our addictions to refined foods precipitate the insulin reaction, but if the shoe fits.

This trail of clues as the cause of obesity is given for one reason, to get my reader to think about his/her own life. This is not written for the person who has no problem keeping their weight under control. This book is for those that struggle with overweight-ism and sugar addiction.

What if the root cause of obesity comes from refined sugars and flours? Would that make a difference in how you looked at food?

It was determined in 2011 by the Statistics on Weight

Counsel that 95% of diets fail, with a 1-5 year window in which people regain their lost weight (16). The diets out there don't want to discuss reality, as you know by the commercials we see from them. Beautiful stars, handsome athletes and proud people of all professions regale us with the virtues of their diets, without telling about the failure rate.

It all sounds so good. You can eat what you want, your favorite foods, showing pictures of sweets and processed flour goodies. The reason they do that is because teaching that those goodies are the exact reason they are having a problem is too tough. By the way, the people giving testimonials may have had to sign a non-disclosure form so that if and when they regain the weight they cannot talk about it.

How do you tell an addict that he/she will have to get off whatever the substance is for the rest of his/her life? You won't make much money with that tactic.

I am a nutritionist. I have people come to me for appraisal of different problems. I cannot diagnose, treat or cure anything. I am not a doctor or nurse. I am a nutritional journalist and counselor, and I love it. There's so much to read and study about the science of nutrition. I can, however, appraise the diets of my clients to help them come into balance.

I have talked with many people whom I will never see again. They are not at the point of recognizing the possibility that they might have an actual addiction. Remember I cannot diagnose, so I discuss the facts we have looked at here today, and I let them draw their own conclusion. The people who draw the conclusion that refined foods may be their problem and take on the task of dealing with a refined foods addiction are successful in their weight loss goals. As long as they follow the advice to the many voices extolling the virtues of refined food abstinence (17), they keep their success going.

As time goes, on this becomes easier and the part of their lifestyle that they would never change. You will not need to think that you will be abstaining forever. There is a place for sugar, refined flour, rice and corn, I promise, but not until you have gotten this addiction under control. I'll tell you about this in a while. First, let's understand the dangers of too much insulin.

Dangers of High Insulin and Insulin Resistance

The consumption of high carbohydrate foods causes overproduction of insulin. So since I am trying to get you to see my way about things let's talk about the dangers of insulin.

Here's a list of the dangers of high insulin taught at a lecture given by Dr. Ron Rosedale, M.D. on August 1999:

- Deficiency of Magnesium (this is particularly bad as Magnesium is required for all energy producing intracellular reactions)
- Stimulation of the sympathetic nervous system (fight or flight)
- Increased risk of heart attacks
- Cardiovascular disease
- Increase levels of triglycerides
- Increased plaque build up
- Increased excretion of Magnesium and Calcium
- Inhibits thyroid function
- Increased fluid retention
- Hormone resistance
- Increased accumulated damage from oxygenation and glycation
- Increased gluconeogenesis (burning muscle for energy)
- Increases the rate of aging (18)

Even hiking the frozen tundra of Canada won't protect someone from eating too many peanut butter cups. In other words, exercise will not stop the damage from too much insulin.

Homeostasis

The body loves and strives for balance. It loves to have equilibrium between all the internal components, despite changes to the environment. This form of stability in our body is called homeostasis. Most often when we are in homeostasis we feel the best.

Magnesium plays a big part in the digestion of foods because it is necessary as a cofactor in enzymes. When a person eats something sugary it will take lots of magnesium to digest that. As a rule, the fruits and vegetables you eat come with the necessary enzymes needed to break down that food. That's why when an apple falls from a tree it will decompose. The apple has the enzymes needed to break down that food. Good thing, because it would be no fun to have to deal with mountains of food that could not decompose and break itself down.

Sugar, on the other hand, has not one enzyme to aid in the process of digestion. It takes a large amount of magnesium to help digest sugar and all of that has to come from our own body. As a result, the stores of magnesium become deficient.

Uh oh, calcium is dependent on magnesium and there is a ratio of calcium to magnesium needed in the blood for things to work. So much magnesium has been used for digesting the sugar you just ate that now that ratio is out of balance.

Calcium and phosphorus are dependent on each other, now they are out of balance. In both cases, the calcium is left out of a correct ratio and causes a toxic calcium effect (19). (It's no wonder people report that when they get off sugar and processed foods they notice a big reduction in tartar, that hard crusty stuff on the back of their teeth. That could be from the reduction of acid in the mouth due to a sugar-free diet. It might also be that minerals in the body are more in balance and not able to deposit onto the teeth from the saliva.)

Phosphorus and zinc work synergistically, now that is out of balance. This goes on and on. The body bravely strives to keep itself in balance and does the best it can.

When the body does not have to deal with processed foods, it is much easier to feel the great feeling of being in balance and in homeostasis.

Reserve Cells

The human body has in its wonderful make up something called reserve cells. Reserve cells give the body and its respective organs the ability to perform in extraordinary ways.

Then one day the reserve cells become used up. Yep, all gone, and what is left is the bare necessities to keep life going. If you keep up your destructive behavior then you start to destroy the skeleton crew that is left.

Take the pancreas for instance. For years the sugar addict stresses the pancreas each time they eat high amounts of sugar, causing cell die off. Remember that eating refined foods that are high in carbohydrates is like having the pancreas being kicked by a metal toed-boot. The pancreas was never designed to cope with that much sugar. As time goes on we are left with that skeleton crew of cells that are keeping us going. As those die off, our bodies start to malfunction.

Just like the ship that loses its last remaining sailors, those ones who keep the engines running, we lose the cells that produce the insulin we need and high blood sugar becomes a real problem. So much so that we now have pre-diabetes, Type 2 Diabetes, then full blown insulin dependent Type 1 Diabetes with all its damaging effects.

There are so many that deal with Type 1 Diabetes and it is difficult. Then there are the ones that are developing Type 2 Diabetes and they really do not realize what is happening until it is too late. Usually, a change of diet and exercise will greatly help the problem but I contend that controlling the sugar and processed flour addiction will, to a great extent, eliminate the problem of Type 2 Diabetes.

There is a need to help people recognize what the real problem is. It is processed sugar and processed flours. That is the problem and they are the evil ones. There I said it.

We just ran through the dangers of insulin and insulin resistance and we know that sugar creates those problems. Now let's look at the other dangers of sugar.

Sugar Dangers

A pioneer in the dangers of sugar consumption is Nancy Appleton. She wrote *Lick the Sugar Habit* and *Commit Suicide by Sugar*. She has a blog "Nancyappleton.com" which everyone should visit just so you can read her list of "141 Dangers of Sugar (just kidding, it's 144)". There is exhaustive research done on these claims. I'd like to mention here a few of the notable dangers from her list.

- Sugar can cause premature aging.

- Sugar can cause anxiety, inability to concentrate and crankiness in children.

- Sugar interferes with the body's absorption of calcium and magnesium.

- Sugar intake increases advanced glycation end products

- Sugar can lead to alcoholism.

- Sugar assists the uncontrolled growth of Candida Albicans (yeast infections).

- Sugar can decrease the amount of growth hormones in the body.

- Sugar lowers enzymes ability to function.

- Sugar can cause headaches, including migraines.

- Sugar can contribute to Alzheimer's disease.

- Sugar can cause asthma.

- Sugar increases the chances of getting irritable bowel syndrome.

- Sugar can affect central reward systems.

- Sugar can cause cancer of the rectum.

- Sugar can cause renal (kidney) cell cancer.

- Sugar can cause liver tumors.

- Sugar plays a role in the cause and the continuation of acne.

- Sugar can ruin the sex life of both men and women by turning off the gene that controls the sex hormones.

- Sugar can cause fatigue, moodiness, nervousness, and depression.

- Sugar can make many essential nutrients less available to cells.

- Sugar can lead to higher C-peptide concentrations.

- Sugar causes inflammation.

- Sugar can cause diverticulitis, a small bulging sac pushing outward from the colon wall that is inflamed.

- Sugar can decrease testosterone production.

- Sugar impairs spatial memory.

- Sugar can cause cataracts.

- Sugar is associated with higher rates of chronic bronchitis in adults.

I have included these so that my reader will grow in appreciation of the fact that sugar is malicious in many ways. Generally speaking, the dangers of sugar consumption pertain to most of us, but these dangers warrant a little deeper explanation.

Premature Aging

The first one listed is 'Sugar can cause premature aging'. That's a big one. Scientists estimate that human lifespan should and could be around 120 years. The average lifespan in 2017 is 79 years (20). There is a Chinese proverb that says most Men dig their graves with their teeth. (21) They were so very wise.

It seems that sugar which creates high insulin is definitely implicated in most of the symptoms of aging.

Dr. Rosedale, M.D. informs the public in his speech on Aug. 1999 at the Designs for Health Institute's Boulder Fest Seminar this, "We found in animal studies that the rate of aging can be largely controlled by insulin, but the damage that accumulates during that aging is caused largely by sugar".

Glycation

Glycation is not understood as well as it should be. Sugar is a sticky molecule and has an unhealthy attachment to protein. When sugar molecules contact a protein in our body called collagen, it produces an enzyme that actually breaks down the collagen which can produce wrinkles as well as the cross-linking that occurs in the collagen causing tissue to be inflexible and ridged (22).

Collagen is found in the skin, bone and connective tissue. Whoa, and sugar is breaking that down. Want to keep your skin young and supple? Eliminate sugars from your diet.

There are other factors of course such as sun exposure and genetics. However, stopping the breakdown of collagen from the inside is enormous.

Glycation increases the stiffness of blood vessels as we age. Atherosclerosis is described as hardening and thickening of the arteries and the usual cause of heart disease, stroke and peripheral vascular disease. Heart disease is still the number one cause of death in the United States. We in the US top the world's sugar consumption by nearly twice the per capita amount (23).

Candida Albicans

Do you have sugar cravings? That is a big indicator of yeast overgrowth. Almost everyone has Candida, which is the name of this malicious fungi. No, I didn't say fun guy! Yeast is indigenous to our intestines and is usually kept in check by the good flora. While it's in the intestines it is a non-invasive sugar-fermenting organism.

However, Candida yeast can change to a fungus like critter. This happens under various conditions but some predominant reasons are:

- eating too much sugar and refined carbs,

- when we are under stress

- when we take antibiotics which kill off the good intestinal flora as well as bad bugs

- when we have nutritional deficiencies

Candida is known to double its population in just one hour under the right conditions. With these right conditions, the fungus form of Candida Albicans is now described as Candidiasis. The yeast turned fungus has rhizoids which are long root-like growths that are very invasive.

The intestines can become porous as the fungus makes its way through the intestinal wall. This is a condition which is referred to as leaky gut. The Candida leaves the gut and becomes dysbiotic (out of the intestines, which is where it should stay). It is now in your blood and is free to cause havoc and mayhem throughout the entire human body, from brain fog to Athletes foot.

We will just talk about brain fog for a minute since so many people that are addicted to sugar have this. There can be many reasons for a foggy brain and bad memory. It can be hormones, not enough sleep, or a poor diet, to name a few. We know for sure that Candida produces a metabolic byproduct called acetaldehyde, among other toxins. This produces brain fog, headaches, nausea and fatigue (24). Well now, that sounds miserable. When you take on a commitment to bring your sugar addiction under control you may also be helping to bring that Candidiasis condition under control.

The sugar cravings may be lessened. Candida is responsible for so many problems. You may find that vast arrays of unpleasant conditions are relieved.

Inflammation

Sugar raises inflammatory markers in the bloodstream. Inflammation has long been shown as a possible cause of arthritis, Alzheimer's disease, anemia, asthma and I'm not even out of the A's yet. The list goes on. Some researchers believe that inflammation is the root of most diseases.

Cancer

Cancer thrives in an acidic environment and sugar is acidic. Also, cancer cells do have insulin receptors. They actually have more than a normal cell by 10 to 12 times. Sugar consumption increases growth in cancer cells by utilizing the ability of insulin to promote growth.

One of the most accurate ways to detect cancer is by using PET (positron emission tomography). A lucky person gets to drink a radioactive-laced sugar drink. Since those cancer cells love sugar so much, they chow it down and those cancer cells light right up (25,26). Ah, the sweet revenge when we can deprive those malignant cells of what they love and use for growth by abstaining from sugar and refined foods.

Immune System

Our immune system depends on the action of phagocytosis to clean up the blood. Phagocytosis is when white blood cells go around munching on bacteria and other pathogens.

Researchers have found that sugar consumption depresses the process of phagocytosis by as much as 50%, and this effect lasts for hours after sugar is consumed (27).

We invited a young man from Mexico to have dinner with us and when I offered him ice cream for dessert he refused, stating that he was getting a cold and was aware that he should not eat sugar as that would encourage the illness. The culture of the United States of America says when someone gets sick we should take them cinnamon rolls! This shows our lack of knowledge about the dangers of sugar generally and especially the damage it does to our immune system.

Refined Flour, Rice and Corn

Along with the sugars, we need to pick on refined flour, rice, and corn for a while. Throughout this book I have identified sugar as the culprit for our modern day addiction. Truth be known, anything that provokes an insulin response is also part of the problem. Without the fiber, refined flour goes through the intestines so quickly that it raises the blood sugar releasing the insulin reaction that primes the nucleus accumbens, causing cravings just the same as sugar.

Refined flour does no good for the intestines either. Do you remember as a kid when you wanted to make a piñata? You would use white flour and water for the glue and would saturate the paper strips in this gooey stuff. Then you wrapped it around a balloon and could make neat creations when it dried hard and stiff. I can only wonder what kind of glue like sludge it leaves in the intestines, making it hard for the very small villi of the intestines to absorb nutrients from the food we eat.

White refined flour has only been around since the turn of the 20th century. What a success this new technology was. It was discovered how to take the bran and germ away from the wheat kernel in a cost effective way. This meant refined flour could be mass produced.

White flour made everything light and fluffy. *Better Homes and Gardens* ran ads on how your family would really rave about these new baked goods. White refined flour was now a staple in every American home.

We had come a long way. Now wheat, which had been the staple for so much of the human existence, full of fiber, rich in vitamins, minerals, and protein was depleted and processed into a white, non-nutritional powdery substance. After wheat flour is processed what is left is starch and a scant amount of protein.

The nutrition that white flour contains is from supplementation. It was in the 1940's that white bread became enriched. As today, B vitamins, iron, and folic acid were added to white flour (28). Otherwise, any nutrition, beyond calories in the form of carbohydrates and some minor amounts of incomplete protein, is negligible.

What we do know is that refined flours create an insulin reaction which may do a great job of releasing cravings (29) and the "Monster Within".

Refined rice has a similar story to refined wheat. The husk, bran, and germ are removed through an industrial process. When the rice is polished, to give it a white shiny surface, most of the vitamins and minerals are removed. What is left is starch which is turned to glucose in the blood. This raises the blood sugar and causes an insulin spike. Hello, cravings!

Cornmeal is higher on the glycemic index than white sugar. This means it raises blood sugar levels higher, with a corresponding raise in appetite.

Corn is the staple food in Mexico, served at just about every meal. Diabetes has surfaced as the number one killer of women and the number two killer of men in Mexico since 2000, so says epidemiologic researchers.

Our biggest tool in reducing cravings and controlling a sugar addiction is to eat foods that do not spike the insulin. Therefore, white refined flours, rice, and corn can be left to enjoy after the eighteen-month initial commitment, and then eaten with a plan in mind.

MSG

What an amazing day it must have been when the food industry discovered that Monosodium Glutamate (MSG) and it's most potent element, Glutamic Acid, actually caused customers to come back for more.

It was discovered in 1908 by Kikunae Ikeda, a Japanese chemist at the Imperial University of Tokyo. He was researching the seaweed added to food for centuries that made it taste so good. He discovered it was L-glutamine.

This discovery was brought to the American cuisine as "Accent" in the form of Glutamic acid and for pennies made food more delicious. Without adding anything else food tasted more savory and appetizing. MSG is actually a white powder that dissolves rapidly in the mouth and is tasteless, but when added to food the food acquires an amazing flavor, leaving the desire for more.

Obesity is linked to MSG in very direct ways. It has the ability to alter the mind and body, even though it is added as a flavor enhancer.

Here is how it works. On the tongue there are five different flavor detectors, the first four you probably know, salty, sweet, sour, and bitter. The 5th is less known, it's called umami. This is where we get the taste of "pleasant, savory", which is derived from the Japanese word "delicious" and was discovered by Ikeda. It is where we get the feeling in our mouth of satisfying savory aftertaste. Rather elusive to describe but hard to turn down.

Glutamic Acid also triggers a protein receptor on the tongue that triggers chemical reactions that tell the brain it is getting a bounty of healthy food with high nutritional content. Neither one may be true but the body incorrectly interprets this.

The Hypothalamus tells the brain when we are full. MSG has the ability to trick this part of the brain and keep it from being able to recognizing satiety. We are full but we keep eating past fullness. Isn't this a dandy situation for the food industry? Adam Marcus had an interesting article in "Health News" back in 2011. He recounts that "Scientists have speculated that people may eat larger helpings of food with MSG because it just tastes better. Other evidence suggests that MSG might interfere with signaling systems in the body that regulate appetite. (30)

MSG causes insulin to spike three times higher than sugar when added to food. Clinical Pharmacology related research showing that when we eat L-glutamate our insulin secretion is increased.(31) This is particularly interesting since we know that insulin spikes trigger the endorphin pathway, which is the addiction and pleasure center of the brain. Also, Dr. Russell Blaylock, a neurosurgeon, is quoted as saying "Monosodium Glutamate (MSG) literally stimulates neurons to death, causing brain damage to varying degrees."(32). Kind of scary, really!

The public became aware of MSG a while back and it

seems everyone knows we should not be eating this substance. In response the FDA has allowed the food industry to add MSG under these labels:

- Autolyzed Plant Protein
- Autolyzed Yeast
- Ajinomoto
- Calcium Caseinate
- Caramel coloring
- Citric Acid (when processed from corn)
- Cornstarch
- Dough conditioners
- Dry Milk Solids
- Enriched
- Fermented anything
- Flavoring Seasonings
- Flavors and Flavoring
- Flowing Agents
- Gelatin
- Glutamate
- Glutamic Acid
- Gums
- Hydrolized Plant Protein (HPP)
- Lipolyzed butter fat
- Low or no Fat items

- Malt Extract or Flavoring
- Malted Barley (flavor)
- Maltodextrin
- Milk Powder
- Modified Food Starch
- Monopotassium Glutamate
- MSG
- Natural Chicken
- Natural Flavoring
- Natural Meat Tenderizer
- Pectin
- Protease
- Protein fortified anything
- Protease enzymes
- Protein Fortified Milk
- Reaction Flavors
- Rice or Brown Rice, Syrup
- Sodium Caseinate
- Senomyx (wheat extract labeled as artificial flavor)
- Textured Protein
- Soy Protein
- Soy Protein Isolate or Concentrate
- Soy Sauce or Extract
- Spice

- Stock
- Ultra-pasteurized anything
- Vitamin enriched
- Wheat
- Whey Protein Isolate or Concentrate
- Whey Protein or Whey
- Yeast Nutrients
- Yeast Extract

Food Additives that often have MSG included

- Annatto
- Barley Malt
- Bouillon
- Broth
- Caramel Flavoring
- Carrageenan
- Corn Syrup and Corn syrup solids (33)

The moral of this story is you can pretty well figure that the majority of any fast food, restaurant food, packaged food, processed in any way food, has MSG included.

What do we do to protect ourselves from this? We make our own food. I am really sorry, I know it is hard and sometimes not practical, but things msut change for you now. You will become a priority. For the first time since you were a kid, you are going to do what is best for you. Preparing the majority of your meals yourself puts you in control of what goes into the food you are eating.

You will be eating high quality protein and fats, dairy products (except milk), fresh and cooked vegetables, and nuts and seeds. Sounds like you may become a gourmet cook without even trying! These changes in your life will make overcoming sugar addiction possible. (There are specific guidelines in "The Plan" section.)

It is a change that will enhance your health and wellness for the rest of your life. We only get one body, so overcoming this addiction by eating healthy low carb food is an amazing way to protect and value it.

BMR (Basal Metabolic Rate)

Recently I attended a Dietitians training and had my BMR (Basal Metabolic Rate) tested. This is the rate of calories expended while at rest for a 24 hour period. I was looking over everyone's shoulder checking out their rates. (I'm tall so I can get away with that.)

You may have an understanding that the average calories you can eat for a day are somewhere around 2000. I know that number gets quoted by dieticians a lot. Maybe they want you to like them. I have the hard job of telling you the truth. Only a 6-foot tall man or taller, or an athlete in training has a BMR that high.

The rest of us have to look at the hard facts. One of them is that the BMR for men and women slows down 5% to 10% every 10 years after the age of 20 to 30. Also, without some effort, we can become more sedentary as we age.

Women have a lower BMR than men by about 10%. BMR also is determined by how much body fat and muscle mass a person has.

Women typically have a higher percent of body fat with a lower percent of muscle than men. This translates to men having a higher BMR to maintain that muscle. This partially accounts for why men lose weight easier than women. Women that are leaner and/or strength train and are physically active will have a higher BMR.

Body fat insulates the body and makes it easier to keep the body core temperature. The temperature of a persons' environment will also affect BMR. The body will strive to keep our temperature at an average of 98.6, except at night when the body temperature typically decreases. (This is why it is such a great idea to stop eating at 7pm, as during sleep we use the least amount of calories.) Anything that changes our body temperature during the day, either higher or lower, will cause the body to work at achieving its optimal temperature and that will raise the BMR.

The size of a person's body mass will reflect on his/her BMR. The larger and taller a person is the higher the BMR will be to sustain organ function and temperature. As a person loses weight their BMR will decrease.

There are a few different equations to figure out a person's BMR and their answers only vary by about 50 calories. You can find them on apps and on the internet. Just to make it easy, I have included a chart of BMR for the average person. The closer you are to your goal weight, the lower BMR you will choose in your category. Also age will have a bearing.

This is the average, so you can make some adjustments, but this fact is true: without purposeful intervention, the older you get the lower the BMR goes. In other words, if you don't exercise as you age your BMR decreases. You may ask, "So, OK, if I exercise, then my BMR will be much higher and I can eat sugar, right?" Funny sugar addicts! (The answer is NO in case you weren't sure.)

Be careful with thinking you can raise your caloric intake. Even though exercise is recommended to increase one's BMR, experts say that exercising causes the appetite to increase, offsetting the benefit of the calories expended. Researchers are finding that after vigorous exercise, we tend to be lazier through the rest of our day. So we are hungrier and more tired. Have you ever wondered why you can't maintain those pounds you took off even though you exercise? Well there it is. This is why it is essential to use your BMR to gauge how many calories you take in each day.

Choosing the average or mean BMR will work for most people to start out. There is about a 200 to 400 calorie variance between the low and the high of the amount of calories you can eat. Try to stay within the this range.

It's not always possible to hit the mean amount of calories in a day but if you stay within the range you should do great.

Basal Metabolic Rate

Men

Height	Range	Mean
5'4"	1200-1600	1400
5'5"	1275-1685	1480
5'6"	1340-1750	1550
5'7"	1410-1820	1610
5'8"	1480-1890	1680
5'9"	1550-1960	1750
5'10"	1615-2030	1815
5'11"	1685-2095	1885
6'0"	1750-2165	1950
6'1"	1820-2235	2020
6'2"	1890-2300	2100
6'3"	1960-2370	2160
6'4"	2030-2440	2230

Basal Metabolic Rate

Women

Height	Range	Mean
5'1"	1120-1350	1240
5'2"	1135-1370	1255
5'3"	1155-1390	1275
5'4"	1195-1430	1315
5'5"	1235-1470	1355
5'6"	1270-1500	1390
5'7"	1310-1550	1430
5'8"	1350-1585	1470
5'9"	1370-1600	1490
5'10"	1410-1650	1530
5'11"	1450-1685	1570
6'0"	1490-1730	1610
6'1"	1530-1970	1750

Calorie Consumption

When the weight is in the normal range it is much easier to go for an evening stroll or to take the stairs. Taking off the extra pounds makes life so much easier in every way. To facilitate this we will want to keep the calories in a correct range for our size, BMR, age, and activity level. That is why some diet plans out there fail in the long run. Calories do count. (#@$%&###. I just swore.) It's no fun for calories to count, especially if it causes us to feel deprived.

So what will help with that feeling of deprivation? We'll talk about that right after we talk about calorie consumption and exercise, I promise.

But first, this leads us into how many calories should I plan on for weight loss and for maintenance. For weight loss, the average person can take his/her BMR and reduce that by about 200 calories. For maintenance the average person can add about 200 calories a day. So for a woman who is 5'6, this would give her a weight loss calorie consumption of about 1200 calories a day. Then for maintenance she can plan on about 1600 calories a day. If she is a total couch potato then keep it at the BMR of about 1400 calories a day.

Everything is a variable, age, sex, activity, and exercise. You are aiming for a 2 pound loss a week. This of course will vary wildly with each person. Men have it so much better than women in this regard as their weight loss can easily be twice that of a woman and they get to consume more calories. I am going to blame it on a larger muscle mass and testosterone.

We want a consistent loss. Things will vary, but too fast of a loss can be devastating. While I was in a nutrition class in college, we studied the mental effects that have been observed from people losing weight too fast. Depression, anorexia, bi-polar, and even schizophrenia disorders have occurred. On a lesser note, the skin could become saggy, emotions can change due to hormonal imbalances, muscle can be lost decreasing metabolism and strength, and the list goes on.

I believe it is very important to keep weight loss at a moderate pace for safety's sake.

There are so many variables, that is why an important part of the program is to measure yourself. This will be outlined in the "Measuring" section. Record the measurements, but only the first time that you weighed and then not again until the week that you did not lose anything or maybe gained. You will see the inches lost, and that is so important to realize the improvements you have made. It keeps you motivated.

After becoming aware of the calories of food, calorie counting will not be a burden. It will not take long and you will be able to easily judge how many calories you are consuming. There are many internet sites, or apps to put on your phone that will help you keep track. In the search bar of your app store type in calorie counter and you can take your pick. Most are free.

Exercise

Exercise is beneficial on a number of levels so let us take a look at some of the ones that pertain to those troubled by the "Monster Within."

Exercise is almost a must for solving the problem of insulin resistance. Physical activity allows the body to use the glucose already in the cells for energy. When that reserve is used up then the cells will once again be in a position to receive glucose. If the cells feel they are not getting enough glucose then they will put those additional insulin receptors out there.

What a cool side effect of exercise. It can help a person control and reduce insulin resistance. Exercise can also create strong muscles and bones, and keep you limber and able to move more youthfully. Exercise relieves tension and anxiety that comes with this mortal life, reducing depression as well.

Not the least of the benefits is the increase in metabolism a person will experience. Exercise should not be to work off the calories from the cookies you ate yesterday. Please review the section on the dangers of high insulin. Exercising does not negate the damage done by having a high level of insulin in the blood. Not unless you are eating the high carb stuff at the same time you are exercising. And no, it is not a good idea to eat junk food while you exercise. Addicts think like that you know.

I watched a documentary once that showed a middle-aged lady preparing for her trek across the Canadian frozen tundra. She was walking and she was going alone. As I was watching her, I was trying to figure out her goal in doing this. Was it to be the first person to do this? No, others have done that. Was it to increase her stamina? She did not express that. Was it for the adventure of it? That trek looked hard and boring.

It was when she displayed her provisions she was taking that it all came to light. Her food for the entire trek was a large plastic bag, maybe the 55-gallon size, filled with peanut butter cups, unwrapped and ready to eat. Ok, now it made sense. She was going to be able to eat all the chocolate peanut butter candy her little heart desired. And she could honestly tell everyone she needed those calories for the energy.

I believe in moderate exercise, just enough to keep the cardiovascular in good shape and the muscles toned and strong. That will be different for each person as so many people are not fans of exercise, or maybe it is the opposite. Vigorous exercise can give a person an adrenaline rush that will initiate an endorphin pathway response. They can literally get high on exercise.

You may think this is a great addiction to have. You get that feel good, happy feeling while being in great shape.

With all addictions, there is a cost. Research is showing that those who participate in an exercise that is physically very demanding show signs of declining vitality rather that an increase in health.

An example would be marathon running, where there is 7 or more hours' duration of demanding training each week.

Marathon runners probably feel that they get picked on for their tenacity. I do admire long distance runners, they are to be praised in many ways. However, there is one thing that can be highlighted that may be helpful. There is a chemical found in the blood of marathon runners, after their completion of a 26-mile run, called Troponin. It is found in these runners without exception.

Troponin is produced when there is a death of the cardiac muscle, the same as in a heart attack. This level of physical activity causes micro-tearing to the heart muscle. The experts are still trying to figure out how much running is good and how much is detrimental. Some experts are saying that you can maximize the benefits at 2 to 3 hours of running a week. James H. O'keefe, MD, director of preventive cardiology at the Mid America Heart Institute at St. Luke's Health System in Kansas City is quoted as saying in the *Mayo Clinic Proceedings,* "Healthier exercise patterns involve not such extreme duration or intensity".

The exercise you do should not leave you always feeling exhausted, the feeling that you want to go to bed for the afternoon. There will be other things to look for when you become too stressed from over-exercising. Do you feel depressed, do you have trouble sleeping, for women, has your menstrual cycle changed, do you feel anxious or moody, do your joints hurt? When beginning an exercise regime it's normal to feel a little tired, stiff, and sore, but this should wane with a little time and you should begin to feel more energetic with an enhanced feeling of well-being. If we are lucky we will get to grow old in these bodies, and it will go better for us if we don't wear them out.

Do not get me wrong. I am not giving you a pass on exercise. Dr. Carl Lavie, who was also involved in the running study at St. Luke's, makes it clear in his statement, "People who exercise do better than people who don't exercise." The benefits of appropriate exercise certainly out-weigh the negatives and will give life-long dividends.

I am a big fan of weight lifting, even if you start out using soup cans for weights, in front of your favorite TV show. Weight training will increase your muscle mass, shape and tone the body, and give you strength when you need it.

Weight lifting will strengthen the fast twitch muscle fibers which are the ones responsible for quick movements. The ability to move quickly will decline as we age if we neglect this component of our body.

It's recommended by experts to start any weight training with a 10-minute cardio warm up, then lift weights with a particular muscle group in mind. For example, one day can be for strengthening the upper body and back, with the next session on another day to focus on lifts that strengthen the legs and gluts. Follow with stretching to stay limber.

Variety in your exercise is the key. It's called cross training. Athletes train in multiple sports to be able to improve on their main sport.

For the rest of us, cross training gives the average person improved fitness overall without the wear and tear that comes from participating in only one activity. Any movement that is done repeatedly can cause problems. If a person did only squats then the quadriceps, that muscle on the front of the thighs, would become stronger than the other supporting muscles. The hamstrings, the muscles on the back of the thighs, are the opposing muscles to the quads, and if the hamstrings are neglected, they will be weaker and this imbalance can cause injury.

It also causes stress and inflammation to the area that is repeatedly worked. Break up your workouts by offering variety to your body. For example, alter weight training with a day of just walking, then a day where you do stretching such as Yoga, then go for a bike ride, then back to your weight lifting routine. You will get to all the muscle groups that way, and give a needed break to any areas in question.

We need to try and keep the Basil Metabolic Rate (BMR) up for many reasons but maintaining and increasing muscles which create a higher BMR seems sensible. Keep in mind that the body is designed for constant movement with periods of rest. Enjoy those periods of rest but keep on moving!

Now here's that lifeline I promised you on not feeling deprived.

The Skinny on Fats

What takes away that feeling of hunger and deprivation? You can do this by eating enough of the good fats.

Fat helps you feel full and satiated. Remember that person who was eating until she was full and could not stop? When you eat fat the body produces a hormone called CCK, cholecystokinin. It is what is responsible for the sick feeling you get when you eat fat. When you eat enough fat and then more, you feel like you could up-chuck, right? Well, you could. CCK will cause vomiting if more fat is ingested than the body can process. So you stop eating and are happy to do so.

Carbohydrates have no such stop valve. You can eat and eat until you pop and then are sorry you have to quit. It works well for our survival mechanism as continued carbohydrate consumption means more Hmg CoA reductase which means more fat produced and stored. However, this is not good for weight loss goals.

So much confusion on fats! They cause heart disease, right? That's what we keep getting told. Here's the truth as we know it in 2017. There is no research anywhere that links cholesterol and cardiovascular disease. None that are not sponsored by a pharmaceutical company. The fact is we have a biological need for fats. The outer cell membrane of every human cell is actually composed of fat. Our brains are 60% fat! (34) (It is a relief to know that we are all fatheads, not just me!)

We need fat for insulation and energy, for producing hormones, and for structure and support of our organs. However, there are good fats and bad fats.

Good Fats

Saturated Fats: butter, cheese, chicken fat, coconut oil, dairy cream, eggs, sour cream They are called saturated because they have no double bonds between carbon molecules as they are saturated with hydrogen molecules. They are typically solid at room temperature. It used to be thought that saturated fat could only be used for energy. This is quickly becoming a myth of the past.

Dr. Mercola is a *New York Times* best-selling author, and has a newsletter that I recommend everyone visit. He lists on his website "Mercola.com" as of September 22, 2009, these benefits of saturated fats:

1) Improved cardiovascular risk factors

> Saturated fat plays a key role in cardiovascular health. The addition of saturated fat to the diet reduces the levels of a substance called lipoprotein (a) that correlates strongly with risk for heart disease. Research has shown that when women diet, those eating the greatest percentage of the total fat in their diets as saturated fat, lose the most weight.

2) Stronger bones

> Saturated fat is required for calcium to be effectively incorporated into bone. According to one of the foremost

research experts in dietary fats and human health, Dr. Mary Enig, Ph.D., there's a case to be made for having as much as 50 percent of the fats in your diet as saturated fats for this reason.

3) Improved liver health

Saturated fat has been shown to protect the liver from alcohol and medications, including acetaminophen and other drugs commonly used for pain and arthritis.

4) Healthy lungs

For proper function, the airspaces of the lungs have to be coated with a thin layer of lung surfactant. The fat content of lung surfactant is 100 percent saturated fatty acids. Replacement of these critical fats by other types of fat makes faulty surfactant and potentially causes breathing difficulties.

5) Healthy brain

Your brain is mainly made of fat and cholesterol. The lion's share of the fatty acids in the brain are actually saturated. A diet that skimps on healthy saturated fats robs your brain of the raw materials it needs to function optimally.

6) Proper nerve signaling

Saturated fats, particularly those found in butter, lard, coconut oil, and palm oil, function directly as signaling messengers that influence metabolism, including such critical jobs as the appropriate release of insulin.

7) Strong immune system

Saturated fats found in butter and coconut oil (myristic acid and lauric acid) play key roles in immune health. Loss of sufficient saturated fatty acids in white blood cells hampers their ability to recognize and destroy foreign invaders, such as viruses, bacteria, and fungi.

I think it is safe to say that saturated fats are our friends. Here are a few more fats that are beneficial as well:

Monounsaturated fats: {theses can be used for cooking} olive oil, peanut oil, almond oil, avocado oil, and hazelnut oil.

Polyunsaturated fats: {these fats should not be used for cooking as heating damages them} Safflower oil, unprocessed corn oil, nuts, seeds, and salmon.

Essential fatty acids: (primrose and borage), Sesame seed oil, wheat germ oil, and fish oils

MCT Oil: MCT stands for medium chain triglycerides and is derived from coconut oil. Because of the structure of MCT's they have a unique ability. They can cross the intestinal membrane without being digested. The liver takes MCT and quickly turns it into ketones that can be used for energy. It has no flavor so you could eat it off the spoon or in some green tea in the morning for some quick energy. It is not recommended to cook with MCT as it has a low boiling point.

If you would like to try adding MCT to your daily regime, start slowly as it can have some gastrointestinal issues such as gas, bloating or diarrhea. Also check with your doctor if you have any liver concerns before starting with MCTs.

Bad Fats

The fats to utterly avoid are trans-fats, which in their manufactured form are hydrogenated and partially hydrogenated fats. You'll find these in most baked goods such as commercially produced cakes, cookies, pie crusts, snacks, refrigerator dough, nondairy coffee creamers, margarine and in some peanut butters. The oil used to deep fry french fries, doughnuts and fried meat can also contain transfat from the oil used to fry the food. Trans-fats, hydrogenated and partially hydrogenated fats, are the bad fats. They have been chemically treated at high temperatures to produce a longer shelf life.

We do not have the necessary enzymes to break a trans-fat down so it can be used for energy. Hence, trans-fats become a nuisance bumping around inside of us causing damage. They have nowhere to go as it can't be broken down. Recently some experts have said that it is possible that coronary artery disease comes from not only the free radical damage produced by trans-fats etching the insides of our vascular system which precipitates clogged arteries (35), but also from the thickening that occurs from trans fats lodging themselves in the arterial walls. If trans-fats can't be broken down and used or eliminated, they will go somewhere.

Canola, grape seed oil, and corn oils are in a category by themselves because of the way they are processed. Canola oil is rapeseed. The name Canola oil stands for Canada oil as this is where the scientists were when they devised a procedure to turn this industrial oil into cooking oil. Canola, grapeseed, and corn oil are put through a highly unnatural manufacturing process, using toxic hexane solvent and high heating processes. Since they are polyunsaturated fats, and that type of fat is damaged at high heats, I leave it to the reader to decide if they want these in their diets. The exception would be if these oils were cold pressed or expeller pressed.

Next, I will make good on that promise to help you not feel deprived.

Keto Bombs

Just typing out the words "Keto Bombs" makes me happy! These are sweet treats with lots of fat and are delicious. Yes I said sweet. They are sweetened with stevia, erythritol and xylitol. Any of the said sweeteners would work alone, however a blend of all three seem to negate any side effects of flavor. Also xylitol can cause bloating, gas, and or diarrhea in some people, but blending it in with stevia, and erythritol seems to help that. If it does cause problems, introduce xylitol slowly until your tummy can adjust.

Xylitol is granular like sugar, but sometimes I can feel that granular texture in the completed product. It works great to blend the white granular powder into the consistency of powdered sugar and then blend in the stevia and erythritol. You may want to keep a container of the blend ready for when you are in the mood for something sweet. Keto bombs are very satiating because of the high fat content. Fat helps a person to feel full and that helps control appetite.

The recipe that I have devised mimics a peanut butter cup, an all-time favorite of many of my clients. You can go to the internet and type in "Keto Bombs" and be ready for some delicious and interesting ideas. They are great and should be part of the first week, and then for the time you will be counting calories and achieving weight loss, then just keep on using them for maintenance. Keto Bombs truly take away the feeling of deprivation and can get you through some tough times. It's also a great way to increase your intake of healthy fats.

Keeping the Keto bombs in the fridge gives it a fudge texture. They do melt at room temperature.

Chocolate Peanut Butter Keto Bomb

(Approximately 100 calories for a one-inch square cube)

Ingredients:

2 cups Peanut Butter (Adams, or whatever old fashioned that is sugar-free, Chunky or Creamy)

2 cups coconut oil

8 Tbs sweetener Blend *

Heat the Peanut butter and Coconut oil in the microwave or double boiler until liquid, then add the sweetener and mix well. I use a hand blender.

Pour 1 ½ cups into another bowl. To the remaining mix add

6 Tbs cocoa

6 Tbs sweetener or to taste

Mix well.

Into an 8X10 pan add half of the cocoa mix and put into the freezer until solid. This doesn't take very long. Then add the Peanut Butter mix and put back into the freezer till solid. For the last level add the remaining Coca mix and again put into the freezer until solid. This can be left in the freezer or the fridge, depending on how you like it.

I leave it in the freezer as I like that solid texture, put in the fridge it will be softer, however if left at room temperature it will melt.

Sweetener Blend

Mix equal parts of stevia, erythritol and xylitol. This mix can be stored and you are ready for a great sweetener whenever needed. (tip: blend the xylitol to a powdery consistency to avoid a granular texture)

Be Happy

We love to have pleasure in our lives. The sad truth is that too much pleasure will usually be harmful in one way or another. Consider a drug of choice, particularly sugar and refined foods, we know it is harmful.

When we abstain from these faux foods what can replace or help to replace the pleasure that we get from them? I have a program outlined in this book, and it it for people who are serious about "Taming the Monster Within". The program lasts for eighteen months. There is a common statement I hear with regular frequency from people who are pondering giving up refined foods and sugar for eighteen months. It goes like this, "I might as well die if I can't eat the foods I love, that will be the end of all happiness". It is not the end of happiness. Really!

When people take on this eighteen month challenge he/she will find that they have more time to pursue other things in life. A sugar addiction (this includes refined foods) schedules a person's life for them. You will be unconsciously planning your day around your hit. Will you go to town around lunchtime so you can get that #7 at your favorite fast food place? You will exercise and eat a low carb lunch so you can make a big batch of cinnamon rolls or buy your favorite cake and ice cream for dessert.

Life really is too short to spend so much of our time and energy to appease this addiction. Each person is an individual of course, but would you have more time for other activities that have lasting benefits if you did not have to spend time in the day wrapped around a sugar and/or refined flour addiction?

Let's talk about a few ideas that can help boost your happiness quota. Getting enough sunshine is a big one. Sunshine is a treatment used to treat Seasonal Effective Disorder. The minute we get out into the sunshine our brains start to produce more serotonin. That is the feel-good hormone. Some people are born with a tendency to have a low amount of serotonin produced in their brains. Serotonin regulates anxiety, happiness, and mood. It's thought that a deficiency of this hormone can cause depression. 5HTP which stands for 5 Hydroxytryptophan, is the precursor to serotonin. I like this supplement because it does not take over your body's ability to produce the needed hormone, it just gives the body what it needs to be able to do it itself. Along with this, you may want to try St. John's Wort. This is an herb that is a serotonin uptake inhibitor. That means it keeps the serotonin circulating in the brain so it can continually be used. The synapses of the brain like to take up the serotonin and hold onto it, which causes a lack of its potential. If you are taking anti-depression medication or you suspect your medication is an MAO inhibitor you must stay under the care of your doctor. St. John's Wort is known to interact with some medications. Do not try and medicate yourself as that can have negative side effects. As always, please talk to your doctor first before you do anything that can affect your health in any way.

A group of scientists did research about how art creativity stimulates the ventral striatum of the brain. This part of the brain includes the nucleus accumbens. That is the pleasure center of the brain. Their findings, which they published in *Neuroimage*

(36), show that creativity causes humans to be more engaged in life, resulting in more pleasure, thus happier. Coloring books are very popular now and that would be easy to get started. You may find that starting easy helps to foster this ability. Get some nice colored pencils with sharp tips and the coloring book of your choice.

Creativity comes in many forms. You may want to try your hand at woodworking, sewing, or graphic art. Photography is very popular. Don't make it too difficult at first as that may cause unhappiness!

You can set rewards for yourself when you have achieved different benchmarks. Perhaps when you complete your first week, or when you've accomplished getting your appetite under control. That deserves a massage, or a facial, or whatever would be fun for you. Are you thinking that is too indulgent or expensive? Consider the cost you have paid in your life to have a sugar addiction. A facial is cheap compared to diabetes.

Exercise is proven to boost endorphins and lift the mood. How great is that? You get in shape and get happy at the same time!

Eat more chocolate. (Surprised you didn't I) Sugar-free hot chocolate made with almond milk, some cream, cocoa, and sweetener. Try my chocolate peanut butter keto bombs. Check out the chocolate keto bombs on the internet. Having some chocolate every day makes almost everyone happier!

Everyone likes to feel good about the way they look. My goal for you is to become addiction free and to love yourself and to love life.

This next idea may come as a surprise, however, it is part of our happiness quotient for the day. Chewing!

I have noticed that many sugar addicts are in a big hurry to get their food eaten. They are in such a hurry that they do not really chew their food. It is now known that this habit can increase anxiety and tension. Emily Rosen, Director of the Institute for the Psychology of Eating, writes "Chewing is an important outlet for tension." (37)

When the food goes down without proper chewing, it puts a stress on the body that can cause a sympathetic nervous system reaction. This means that the body goes into a fight or flight situation.

Remember from your high school health class, the autonomous nervous system can respond to a perceived threat to life by stimulating the adrenal medulla. This organ sits on top of the kidneys and it produces hormones that are essential for life, including the hormones that can control our reaction to stress. These hormones are epinephrine, norepinephrine, and cortisol.

Cortisol prepares the body for a fight-or-flight response by flooding the body with glucose, which gives the body an immediate energy source to the large muscles. This makes sense, now you can run away from whatever the threat to life is. Cortisol inhibits the production of insulin because insulin will cause the body to store extra glucose as fat. That won't help you run away, so if you had a tiger chasing you that would be a good thing.

Cortisol narrows the arteries while the epinephrine increases heart rate, which forces our blood to pump harder and faster. We are now in fight-or-flight. Blood flow to the brain and muscles are increased. Sounds a little super human, cool! Hey, wait a minute, we were just trying to eat.

Let's go back to what capacity the body actually has. Chewing our food is supposed to break our food down into a non-recognizable mush. Then, when it goes to the stomach there is further breakdown of the food by the stomachs release of enzymes and acids.

The stomach does have the ability to churn the food which helps to mix these digestive chemicals. We do not have anything that resembles teeth in the stomach. That large scale pulverizing of food has to take place by chewing. When food hits the stomach in large pieces it puts the body into a stressful situation. This is exactly what happens when we are in a hurry to swallow.

The part of the autonomous nervous system we need to work for us when we eat is the parasympathetic nervous system, or as it's commonly known, the rest and digest system. The parasympathetic nervous system is the opposite of fight-or-flight.

It promotes digestion, healing, regeneration, detoxifying, eliminating and building. The parasympathetic nervous system triggers the digestive system to produce all the beneficial enzymes needed to break down food to a form that will help us get the greatest absorption of nutrients.

The mouth releases saliva, the stomach produces HCL, the pancreas excretes digestive enzymes, and the gall bladder releases bile. Well chewed food allows the small intestines to actually get to the nutrients so they can be absorbed.

Swallowing big chunks of food will Initiate the fight or flight system and effectively block all the benefits of rest and digest. The heightened alertness and ability to sprint away are short lived and are followed by cells that are starving for energy since cortisol inhibits the insulin that opens the cells to receive energy.

This hunger in the cells initiates an increase in appetite, so we eat more. And, of course, unused glucose will eventually be stored as fat.

Long term fight-or-flight, with increased levels of cortisol, is known to stimulate fat storage around the belly, cause blood sugar problems, increase anxiety, depression, and insomnia.

What am I getting to? Chew your food so that you cannot detect chunks. How many times will that be? According to the Ohio State University, 5 to 10 times for soft food like fruit, and up to 30 times for pieces of meat.

It is also important to try and eat in a non-stressful environment. Meditate for a moment before you start. For some that will mean saying a prayer over their food, others, just take a breath, smile, and be calm. Dinnertime is not the time to discuss stressful topics. It really is bad for everyone who is trying to eat. The sympathetic nervous system reaction, fight-or flight, is easily initiated. It only takes perceived threats. You don't really need to see a tiger to start that cascade of detrimental hormones. Being scolded for not taking out the garbage will do just fine. Do you watch the news while you eat? I haven't watched a non-stressful newscast in a long time.

Do what you can to encourage the parasympathetic system, rest and digest, while you eat. It should be a time to experience the pleasure of food, and to activate our pleasure receptors through smell and taste. Slow down and commit to sitting at a table for your meal and taking the time it takes to relax and chew thoroughly each bite. It is essential to good health. (Make a little note that reminds you to chew and post it where you can see it when you eat. This principle of good health is easy to forget.)

You surely will find what makes you happy. A dependence on sugar and refined foods as a way to be happy is so temporary, and is followed by a reduction in the pleasure it gives and a regret that increases as time goes by. Find your happiness in something that will bring you joy and satisfaction, something that will foster your continued interest and progression. In my opinion, the principle of happiness is essential to a full, rewarding life.

Dining Out

It's your birthday and your friends want to take you to dinner. You are the guest of honor at your work luncheon or it's your child's graduation and you have reservations at a great restaurant. These kinds of occasions will not stop happening even though you have committed to eighteen months of no refined processed foods. No sugar and no processed flour or white rice. Well, it's ok. You can go to any restaurant out there and have a great meal completely on your plan.

Your cravings and appetite are under control now, so you can make those healthy choices without a problem. At Italian restaurants, choose the salad and steak, chicken, or salmon choice. Instead of the noodles ask for the vegetable of the day. They are usually serving what is in season.

When the bread is brought to the table it is not an issue as that is not what you will be eating for a year and a half, and only then when you have pre-decided. If meth were brought to the table you would not consume that just because it was served. This is actually the same thing. You have an addiction to something that should never have been put in our diets in the first place, so it is really not a sacrifice any more than abstaining from any other drug of choice. If you are not a smoker then walking by a row of tobacco at the grocery store means nothing to you and this is how it is when you are not eating these dangerous and damaging pseudo foods.

Perhaps your group is going to the local "all you can eat" pizza place. That is a great place for you. Have the salad bar of course, and then go pick out your favorite pizza. You will be eating the toppings off and since that will be meat and cheese that is high in fat you will feel happy and satiated. Leave the crust on the plate and the waitress will take it away. No problem!

Can you have seconds? Sure, if you are still hungry, go for it. Appetites have a way of becoming normalized when you keep your insulin levels under control by eating low carbohydrate. Because you are eating plenty of fat there is a great feeling of being full that actually controls your behavior. Now when you are full, you stop eating because that feels better than still eating. The CCK kicks in and you will feel nauseated if you eat more fat than you should. Your body will actually be ahead of your head! You feel full but your brain tells you to keep eating. Do not worry, your head will catch up and now that you have the insulin spikes under control, you will have the ability to tell your brain "No, I'm full, and that is that!" You did not over eat even though the restaurant you ate at might have been an "all you can eat" and food is all around you! So cool! You are in control, and it truly is the best place to be.

Fast Food

It is such a pleasure to be able to just drive up to the window of one of your favorite fast food restaurants and order #6, no maybe #4. Guess what? You can still enjoy this pleasure with a few alterations.

You can get that double burger but ask for the low carb lettuce wrap and no ketchup. The restaurant will take your favorite burger and wrap it in lettuce and it is still delicious.

There is no way to fix the French fries so ask for the side salad with a sugar free dressing. Ranch or Caesar dressing works great and you can usually make this trade without cost.

Get the drink but ask for it to be ice water instead. Try adding stevia to your ice water that is flavored with cola, toffee, or lemon flavorings. Keep a bottle of stevia in your vehicle so you can have it for just this purpose. You can find these usually wherever stevia is sold or on the internet. Drinks sweetened with sucralose or aspartame will cause the insulin to spike and make it hard for you to make it through the day.

There is a fast food chain that serves chili. If you like chili, try that with the extra cheese and sour cream to increase the fat content. Salads are great; however, they hide a lot of things not in your food choices and they are hard to eat on the go. The more hardcore addict you are, the more your insulin spikes with a mere serving of dried cranberries or croutons.

Some fast food eateries have great grilled chicken nuggets that are not breaded. Ask for the Ranch dressing as a delicious dip.

You will be able to find things that will work for you and allow you the joy of the drive in. Don't be scared, you've got this!

Snacks

Snacking between meals can be a life saver in the early period of your new lifestyle. If your brain is still trying to catch up to the fact that your insulin levels are in a healthier range, you may start craving something between meals or when you see a fast food chain that was not a planned stop.

It is very handy to have a fat, and protein snack available. Cheese sticks do a nice job as well as some almonds. That will give you the fat and protein you need, as well as some chewing. Macadamias are pretty wonderful too. Full of fat and crunch.

Pack your choice for the day in a baggy and put it where you can easily find it when you are on the go. Also, remember your bottle of water. If you have water to wash down that snack, you will not feel you need a diet or regular pop as you drive by the local gas station.

When you get further into your eighteen months and are closer to your goal weight, you may find that snacks are not necessary. This is fine as well because we need the insulin levels to stay low. Remember that the act of eating stimulates the intestines to send the signal to produce insulin. Insulin puts you in the fat storing mode, so lower levels of insulin through the day will help keep you in a fat burning mode. However, if you need snacks to help you through till the next meal and to keep you honest, snack away. Keep them within your total calorie count for the day.

Fruit

Do you know the technical definition for "getting squirrely"? I see it all the time. It's a condition where people get nervous, squirmy, and disbelieving. They have the look in their eyes that they are ready to bolt! This happens when I tell them that fruit will raise their blood sugar the same as candy. "But fruit is so good for you!" Well, yes it is unless you are a sugar addict.

Consider that chocolate cake with chocolate frosting has a lower glycemic index than watermelon does by about half. The Glycemic index measures how fast the blood sugar is raised by a particular food. For sugar addicts that is useful because it will give you a clue as to how bad the insulin spike will be. The higher the Glycemic Index number the faster the food is digested and the bigger the insulin spike.

Can you live without fruit? Ask an Eskimo. Fruit will be back in your diet in the form of low carb berries as soon as you reach goal weight. The higher carb fruit will be one of those things you choose to eat and which are planned.

I have a client who had 80 pounds to lose. As I discussed the plan and told her about no sugar, she assured me she almost never ate sugar. I asked her if she ate fruit, and yes, she loved fruit and ate it every day. We took the fruit away and the weight melted off her. If you feel you cannot live without fruit, please be aware that is the "Monster Within" talking. It is actually the insulin spike you do not think you can live without, but it is ok. This feeling will pass as you get this addiction under control and you will forget that you ever got squirrely!

Protein

It is widely known that protein is essential to life and good health. We need it for structure, muscle, the immune system, transport, hormones, energy and production of enzymes.

The amount of protein eaten should be tailored to a person's size and muscle mass. Some researchers say that the optimum level is .05 to 1 gram of protein for each pound of bodyweight, some say 1.5 to 2 grams of protein per pound of body weight. There are so many voices. A rule of thumb that works really well for most folks is to eat protein in amounts that are equivalent to the size of the palm of your hand. Bigger people have bigger palms, smaller people have smaller palms.

Since we are not carrying around a scale most days, this is a great gauge. However, take a moment and measure what the size of your palm is in say, ground beef. Make a patty that looks about the same width and thickness as your palm. Then use a scale and measure the patty. How many ounces is that? Four ounces of chicken contains 36 grams of protein, while 4 ounces of lean ground beef provides about 28 grams of protein. The amount of flesh meat that your palm correlates to can be eaten 2 to 3 times a day. Eating a 12-ounce steak at one sitting would only be appropriate if you weighed in at about 450 pounds and where a body builder and /or athlete.

Experts report that heavy protein intake is implicated in so much that is detrimental to our health. High protein intake is hard on the kidneys, causing stress as these organs have to remove more nitrogen, it may cause demineralization of bones, and it has even been associated with an increase in cancer (38).

Nutritionists agree that too much protein can cause gluconeogenesis (production of glucose from protein, either dietary or from muscle mass) which can spike blood sugar levels causing an insulin reaction and unleash your appetite. Therefore it would be correct to say that too much protein can awaken that "Monster Within". Remember, an insulin spike can set the brain up for a hit in the endorphin pathway and cause you to crave high carb foods all day. No fun!

Protein Drinks

Some clients report that protein drinks cause them to start craving carbs. That is because the densely powdered form of protein goes through the digestion so quickly that it will spike the insulin.

This form of protein is not how the body expects to get its most important building blocks. The body recognizes complete protein such as chicken, beef, sea food, pork, eggs, and all the other foods that are in their natural state.

There is a wealth of information out there about the hazards of protein shakes and also the benefits. A fitness trainer can cherry pick the research he wants to support the program promoted. Most of these studies are only done for a short period of time.

As a nutritionist I have to look at what the body's actual ability is. For millennia humans have eaten the types of protein in flesh meats, dairy products, nuts, legumes, vegetables and fruits. This is how humans have developed. However, now humans are not only asking the body to digest a dense protein that is highly processed, but which also contains synthetic vitamins and minerals.

Nutrients in nature work synergistically and most often are found together in natural, whole foods. Nutrients in protein drinks that are not coming from a whole food are isolates. This means they are isolated and are introduced to the body without the supporting nutrients. The artificial sweeteners aspartame, sucralose and sugar alcohols that are in most protein drinks alter the gut flora in negative ways (39).

Some people have used protein drinks with great success. Some come away starving soon after drinking a protein shake. It depends on which protein drink is used and how fast the body metabolizes it. Search for one that is sweetened with stevia, erythritol, or xylitol as these do not cause an insulin spike in most people. However, since everyone reacts differently, and xylitol is known to cause some gastric distress, determine which of these sweeteners works best for you.

Check to see that the nutrients are coming from a vegetable source for optimum absorption.

This next point is very important. The protein drink of your choice needs to have a fiber content that includes insoluble and soluble fiber, in a 3:1 or 2:1 ratio so the digestion process can be slowed down. This may help prevent an insulin spike. If insoluble fiber is overly predominant it may prevent the absorption of some minerals. It is best to have a protein drink with a good balance of insoluble to soluble fiber.

Forms of protein would be whey, soy, pea, or chicken protein. Chicken protein is new to the market and appears to be beneficial in several ways. More research will come out after this book is published, but it looks like chicken protein is non-allergenic, dairy and gluten free, a complete protein, and digestible.

Vegans and Vegetarians

We require protein to carry on with life and metabolic processes, and human protein is made from 20 amino acids. The body synthesizes all but nine of these. The nine that are not produced by the body must be obtained from diet and this is essential, that's why they are called essential amino acids. Flesh meats, beef, chicken, pork and sea food, are complete proteins which mean they have the amino acids, including the essential amino acids, we need to function properly.

Incomplete proteins are those that are lacking some of those nine essential amino acids and therefore need to be combined with other food that will have the complimenting amino acids to give the body the nine that are necessary from our diet.

I have met with vegans who eat no animal products what-so-ever, and vegetarians who eat no flesh meats but have various ideas on dairy products and eggs. They all have different reasons for their dietary choices. Some choose this lifestyle for faith reasons, some for moral reasons and some for health expectations. I respect them all.

I see vegans and vegetarians who do not make an effort to be mindful of their protein intake. Too little can be as bad as too much protein. Decline from lack of complete amino acids is common. B-12 deficiency is always a concern as well as a lack of carnosine.

Carnosine helps reduce glycation, that destructive binding of proteins and sugars, shown to damage connective tissue, create inflammation and cause problems for organs where flexibility is important. Examples of sensitive areas are the heart, kidneys, skin and eyes.

If you are a vegan or vegetarian I recommend you work with a healthcare professional who can help you make the correct choices. The amount and quality of the protein a person gets are too important to leave to chance.

Ketosis

I suspect you are hearing a lot about Ketosis these days and it is a good thing to understand. A definition of Ketosis would be when the body uses Ketones for fuel. Ketones are small fuel molecules produced when fat is used for energy due to fasting or a prolonged low carbohydrate diet. It's a perfectly natural state for the body to be in.

The brain will be as happy to burn glucose for fuel as it will be to burn ketones. This is a good thing from an evolutionary standpoint. Regular meals were not the norm for most of man's history. Our bodies will only store about 12 hours of energy. After that if we were not able to use our fat stores for energy a person would shut down pretty quickly. Muscle can be turned into glucose by gluconeogenesis but that would rapidly waste a person down to nothing. Using our stored fat can give us many days or even months of reserve energy which would prolong life in desperate situations.

It is common for people to mistake Ketoacidosis for Ketosis. They do sound alike. Ketoacidosis occurs when there is an unrestrained, excessive production of ketones in the body due to a severe malfunction. It could happen to a Type 1 diabetic if they don't take insulin.

Ketosis is a desired state for the body. Not only is it a natural process but it delivers some impressive benefits. Burning ketones for energy is a clean type of fuel. Using carbohydrates for fuel produces abundant free radical damage which can be a suspect in many disease processes. You could say it is a dirty fuel.

Mental focus may improve because during ketosis there is a steady supply of fuel to the brain and blood sugar fluctuations are limited. Cancer cells do not have the ability to use ketones for energy or growth (40). Again Glucose is what cancer uses for energy. Cancer cells have been shown to have 10-12 times more insulin receptors than a normal cell. Also, during Ketosis you use fat for energy and thereby lose body fat.

What I have noticed concerning the people I consult with is that ketosis is difficult to achieve. It is called being keto resistant. The body of a person who eats high carbohydrates is programed to burn sugar for fuel. It is a transition that the body will make but it takes time.

Particular enzymes are needed for ketosis that may not have been produced often. It can be very frustrating if a keto resistant person makes ketosis their goal and it does not happen for them in a timely way. The program outlined in "Taming the Monster Within" is more to help people accept and realize that high carbohydrate and refined processed foods were never supposed to be a frequent part of the human diet. In fact, consuming these villains has produced an addicted society that on the whole believes the refined foods that are killing us are their rite of passage.

What humans will benefit and thrive from is a diet composed of natural food, low in carbs, moderate in protein, and high in fat. Living this lifestyle promotes health, self-esteem, a life free from addiction and all that goes with that. If striving for ketosis will help you do that I am all in. If it becomes a distraction, then do not worry about it and just stick to the program.

Intermittent Fasting

I do recommend intermittent fasting whether you are striving for ketosis or not. It is has too many benefits to ignore. When you eat carbs, the body sends a message for the pancreas to produce insulin. Insulin takes the available carbs and puts them into the muscle and the liver in the form of glycogen. Glycogen can be readily turned into energy when the need arises.

If you do not eat, all the available glycogen will be used up after 12 hours. That is all the body can store. After 12 hours the body will start to use fat as energy.

If you stop eating at 7pm and then have an early lunch the next day at 11am, you will have gone 16 hours without eating. That is intermittent fasting. When you can go from 13 to 18 hours without eating, you get all the amazing benefits of fasting.

It is not really that hard because most of those hours are spent sleeping. The benefits of intermittent fasting are well documented. Here's a partial list:

- Lower insulin levels promote Ketosis, the term used describing the process of burning fat for fuel (41)

- Insulin levels drop which helps reduce insulin resistance. (42)

- Growth hormone increases significantly (43)

- Autophagy increases, which is how the body cleanses cellular debris (44)

- Metabolism increases (45)

- Oxidative stress is reduced (46)

- Inflammation is reduced (47)

- Free radical damage is reduced which can prevent premature aging (ibid)

- Intermittent fasting can promote weight loss (48)

- There are studies with animals that show a reduction in cancer and Alzheimer's disease. Further human studies will need to confirm this, however, it looks promising (49)

Fat Fasting

Through this book I have recommended that any program that affects your health in any way should be monitored by a healthcare professional. This Fat Fasting section will outline a technique of losing weight that should only be used by people who are keto resistant and are under the care of their doctor.

If you are losing weight with a low carb program then do not try Fat Fasting. It will possibly cause too severe of a weight loss. I include this technique because it works for people who are keto resistant. However it can cause lightheadedness, headaches, and possibly weight gain for the average person if you take in more than 1000 calories per day.

I don't recommend this to my clients. You will need a doctor to monitor your progress if you think you are in the category where this is helpful. It is recommended by the experts that before you try Fat Fasting you follow a low carb program for about 4 weeks first. Then if weight loss is stalled you may find Fat Fasting a way to speed up obtaining ketosis, which is burning fat for energy.

It is recommended to only follow the Fat Fast for 3 to 5 days. Fat Fasting consists of eating 75-90% fat, 15-20% protein, and 1-7% carbs.

You will want to only eat the best quality fats, and proteins. The carbs will be vegetables. Your doctor may recommend that you take a vegetable source multi-vitamin supplement. Potassium supplements can help with any muscle cramping, but seek the advice of your doctor.

Drink lots of water as it's known that 1 gram of carbohydrates carries with it 3 grams of fluid, so reducing your intake of carbs to such a low level will cause fluid loss. Fat Fasting should be followed by adherence to a low carb program which entails 20-35% protein, 40-70% fat and 10-20% carbohydrates.

Dr. Atkins wrote about Fat Fasting in his book, *Dr. Atkins' New Diet Revolution.* He gave a one day example of what a Fat Fasting day would look like. It goes like this:

2 oz. sour cream, containing 1 tablespoon of caviar (you could use capers)

Served on three or four crisp fried pork rinds

2 deviled egg halves

2 oz. of chicken salad made with triple the usual amount of mayonnaise

1 oz. of chicken, ham, egg or shrimp salad in half an avocado

2.5 oz. of whipped cream, artificially sweetened (use sweetening blend)

You can find menus plans on the internet or on your smart phone.

Supplements

There are many, many, many, (did I say many), supplements on the market to aide in weight loss. I have two that I find particularly helpful without any malicious side effects.

Konjac Glucomannan comes from the root of the Konjac plant which originates in Asia. It is a fermentable and soluble fiber. Konjac has been around and consumed for thousands of years. It has many favorable traits such as it can give you a beneficial cholesterol level(48), it adds bulk to the diet relieving constipation, and it works well in the colon acting as a prebiotic. A prebiotic gets fermented in the colon and actually feeds necessary probiotics which are the good guys in our intestines.

For our purposes it works to create the feeling of fullness. It can be in the form of a powdered fiber, put into a capsule and sold as a weight loss supplement or bought from the "Miracle Noodle" company as a carb free, non-caloric, fat-free noodle or rice.

Konjac holds many times its weight in water making it a great thickener for soups, stews, gluten free gravies and sugar free puddings. I also recommend putting the powder into a salt shaker and sprinkling it over your food. Sprinkle lightly as you would sprinkle salt. You do not want to notice it as you eat. If you do notice it then you have put on too much. This helps with the feeling of satiety with each meal.

When I was a kid, I loved Cream of Wheat cereal. It was such a comfort food, but it has one fatal problem. It is all starch which will be turned into sugar in the blood and will spike the insulin. You can take 1 ½ cups of almond milk, 1 tablespoon cream, 1 teaspoon of konjac, ½ teaspoon of vanilla, and add enough stevia or the recommended sweetener blend to your liking. Blend it until it is a creamy consistency. Heat until warm, and enjoy a filling Cream of Wheat look and taste alike.

If you like rice pudding, take this mixture and add the "Miracle Noodle" rice with some cinnamon. Very nice! When you discover this for yourself you may find it is indispensable in your goal to not be hungry.

A word of warning-the "Miracle Noodle" products will smell like a dirty sneaker when you open the pouch. The pouch will be full of the product and water. Empty the contents into a strainer and rinse with hot water until the smell is gone, about 3 minutes. This is a small inconvenience considering how versatile and filling the noodles are.

I really like the Angel Hair noodle as it works well whenever you would have used angel hair wheat noodles. Try it with your sautéed vegetables, or with chicken alfredo sauce. Konjac creates a fullness that really helps a person get through a long food-less evening.

The second supplement I find so helpful that it sounds too good to be true is Berberine.

Berberine is a natural supplement that:

- helps combat bacteria (50)

- fights protozoa (51)

- reduces parasites (52)

- reduces fungus(53)

- fights depression (54)

- improves memory and learning (55)

- may help treat leaky gut (56)

- has been shown to reduce inflammation (57)

- contains a chemical found in several plants that is anti-cancer (58)

- reduces LDL cholesterol (59).

- lowers blood pressure (60)

- may prevent heart disease (61)

- may prevent Alzheimer's disease (62)

- helps with rheumatoid arthritis (63)

- helps with osteoarthritis (64)

- shows protective abilities for the liver (65)

- helps with ulcerative colitis (66)

- helps inflammatory bowel disease (67)

- anti-viral (68)

- has shown the ability to treat diabetic neuropathy (69)

And this is so fun! Berberine actually activates AMPK activity, and creates new mitochondria (70)

Mitochondria are the little energy factories in our bodies. They create the ATP that our bodies use for energy. Endurance training increases the number of mitochondria in our muscle cells, so when we need it, we can increase our peak performance.

AMPK, or adenosine monophosphate-activated protein kinase, is an enzyme. This enzyme is activated by exercise, which, among other reasons is why exercise is great for us.

AMPK releases energy generating processes such as glucose uptake and fatty acid oxidation and decreases energy consuming processes such as protein and lipid synthesis. It helps us use the sugar in our blood and helps us to burn fat.

This is a wonderful thing for those who have insulin resistance. Berberine improves insulin sensitivity. We can get those incredible benefits of exercise from taking a pill!!!!! Can you see me? I'm doing the Happy Dance!!

With all the helpful supplements out there, it seems logical that this should be the number one supplement you take.

The dose is best when split through the day as the experts say that Berberine has a short half-life. It is recommended by those experts to take 1500mgs a day, so that would be 500mgs 3time a day (71). Always check with your doctor before starting any program that will impact your health in any way.

Feeling Full

One of the "Monster's" favorite tools is the trick to get people to overeat. When there is an insulin spike, the cravings cause a person to think they still need to eat even though they feel full. It may not even be pleasant, but the desire to continue to eat is there. This may be caused by the lowered blood sugar that insulin spikes produce, or the lack of enough protein, fat and fiber in the diet, or both.

As time goes on you will be able to feel when you are full. There are no longer the physical cravings that are caused by the insulin spikes', however, the mental cue to keep eating will linger. It has been part of the programming that goes with a physical addiction.

You have been tricked into thinking that overeating is pleasant. Take a moment to ponder on what full feels like. As time goes on it will be unpleasant to keep eating past satiety. It won't be recreational eating anymore. It will feel more like punishment because it is uncomfortable. The human stomach is about the size of a person's fist. The stomach has the ability to stretch to about 40 times its size so that it can accommodate a large meal or water intake. That is the physical reason you can keep eating after you have started to feel full. After the stomach empties it will reduce back to its original size.

As your eighteen month commitment progresses, your reaction to feeling full will change. Feeling full will be the cue to stop eating, and you can do it now because the "Monster's" incessant cravings are gone and your brain will come to understand and except what feeling full means. You are changing. It will be desirable to stop eating at full.

Remember that person who thought they had no will power and no character? When the insulin spikes are gone, you will see a different person evolve. So many people who talk to me during this transition seem, at first, surprised and amazed with their lack of appetite. Then as time goes on, they gain a confidence that comes with knowledge and experience. They have removed the mask of the "Monster" and revealed where the problem of overeating really came from. And it was not from them.

Water

Once you start eliminating the sugar and processed flours from your diet you will notice that you have to make a trip to the bathroom more frequently. This happens because your body is burning up the extra glycogen that has been stored in your muscles and liver.

Glycogen break down lets the body release a lot of water. Also as insulin levels drop the kidneys start to get rid of this excess water (72).

If you get your water from a reverse osmosis system, make sure to add some colloidal minerals as reverse osmosis not only removes chemicals but minerals as well (73).

It is a great idea to have water by your side so you can be sipping on it throughout the day.

The recommended amount right now from the experts is half an ounce to every pound of body weight. A 120 pound person will do nicely to drink about 60 ounces of water a day. Harvard Medical School published in their *Harvard Health Publications*, Sept. 2016, some great insight on why we need to keep hydrated.

The list includes:

1. carrying nutrients and oxygen to your cells

2. flushing bacteria from your bladder

3. aiding digestion

4. preventing constipation

5. normalizing blood pressure

6. stabilizing the heartbeat

7. cushioning joints

8. protecting organs and tissues

9. regulating body temperature

10. maintaining electrolyte (sodium) balance.

Create the habit of keeping hydrated so you can reap the benefits for the rest of your life.

Green vs Black Tea

All tea is green tea, but to get black tea the tea leaf has been fermented. With that fermenting process comes some new chemicals that are not in green tea.

Theophylline is an important one to know about as the list of malicious side effects are numerous. Experts report that some of these could be nervousness, lightheadedness, fainting, convulsions, pounding or rapid pulse, shakiness, and even seizures. Black tea also has the ability to get you addicted to it which creates the opportunity for an overdose.

I recommend green tea as the benefits are many. One of the benefits for our purposes comes from epigallocatechin-3-gallate or EGCG for short. The great thing about EGCG is that this phytochemical has a thermogenesis component and is a fat oxidizer. It speeds up your metabolism and helps you burn fat. EGCG is not just another pretty face. Researchers are finding benefits for heart disease, hypertension, stroke, as well as hopeful findings for Alzheimer's and Parkinson patients because it promotes neurogenesis. Neurogenesis is the process where neurons are created from neural stem cells and who among us couldn't use a few more neurons?

Get Ready

When you have made that commitment and are ready to start, there are some changes you need to make.

Remove all the carbs that might give you problems. Keep these trouble makers away from your vision and out of your shelves, pantry and fridge.

If you have a hungry mob at your house and you plan on feeding them as usual, do not feel bad about clearing out your cooking space. It is ok to store the cereal away from the kitchen. This is important in the beginning to not court temptation. Remember this is an addiction and you need all the help you can get. You would not ask a recovering alcoholic to make a wine sauce, so do not expect yourself to have to make high carb anything. I do not want you handling it, smelling it, or cleaning up the mess.

Stock Up

Keep the foods you need plentiful and available. That hungry mob will want some too!

Plan your meals early in the day. Do you need meat to be slowly roasting in the oven or crock pot? Start it cooking early in the day. Do you want green beans sautéed in olive oil and pesto? Start that before you actually need it, and just keep it on warm. Make plenty, it's delicious and everyone will appreciate your willingness to share.

Use the Internet. It is abundant with low carb sugar-free recipes. There are low carb sugar-free cookbooks in abundant supply.

Some programs are not sugar, processed flour, and white rice free, but they are sure to offer some ideas that can be converted to your needs.

Use Parmesan cheese to coat your fried chicken. You can also fry some Parmesan cheese and create Parmesan chips. You can do that with multiple cheeses. Mozzarella, Colby Jack, and Cheddar work great.

Cauliflower is such a versatile vegetable. Make it into faux mashed potatoes or cauli-rice. Most recipes for a rice look-a-like come from cauliflower and are generally called cauli-rice. They call for you to grate cauliflower to get it to the consistency of rice. I am always in too much of a hurry so I have discovered it works fine to blend the cauliflower while it is raw. The flavor is bland enough that it lends itself to whatever spices you add.

Buy the ingredients for your sweetener blend so you have it on hand. Keto bombs are so important to help with cravings and the feeling of satiety. I want you to feel happy and satisfied all the time.

Keto diets are very popular and this is a movement that will not be stopped. The new ideas will be out there.

Use the vegetables in season and learn new recipes. This is important because this is not one of those 6-week diets. The "Taming the Monster Within" program will last your lifetime and variety will win the day.

Weigh Day

As you plan this new beginning, pick the day you are going to start. It really does not matter, Mondays are nice but sometimes later in the week is better for some people. This day will be your weigh day. On day one, weigh. It is best done about an hour and a half after you wake up and before you drink. Wear or do not wear the same thing every time you weigh. Only weigh once a week. You will want your happiness and joy to come from making the correct decisions day in, and day out-not dependent on what the scale says. Your weight just gives you an idea of how you are doing.

There will be ups and downs for a variety of reasons. You may have started a new exercise regime which can cause you to hold on to fluid. For example, lifting weights damages the muscle so that it can repair itself and be bigger and stronger. This can cause temporary water retention.

If you are a menstruating woman you could gain 5 pounds during that time. But it could come off in the following week and you may get a 7-pound loss that next week. Maybe you were under the weather, that can cause fluctuations in weight. With so many variables, it really helps not to be too tied to the scale. Stick to weighing once a week on the same day and same time.

Measuring

On the day you have picked to start your new life you will need to measure yourself.

I have included a list of the areas to measure. Make yourself a chart to record these measurements on.

This tool comes in very handy on those days where the scale does not show a loss. Only on the weigh days that you don't show a loss will you measure again. The purpose of this is to see that you are shrinking whether the scale shows it or not. Inches will be gone, oh happy day! That is important on those difficult weigh days, and they will come.

Everyone plateaus. The fat cells do not like to lose their voluptuous curvy sizes. They like big and will hold water until they realize "I guess we really are going to get small". It could take a week or two for the scale to show the weight loss. Stay on the plan and follow the rules no matter what.

I have several clients who lose a half pound a week. It is not the 2 pounds a week we are going for; however, it is regular and consistent so that makes me happy. I remind them not to be in too much of a hurry because they have a year and a half, remember? Eighteen months will give them plenty of time to reach goal weight and learn how to maintain.

At the end of our time together you will be where you want to be; not afraid of any social gathering, any dinner out on the town, or any sugars and processed foods being served anywhere, anytime. You will always have the addiction; however it will not have you. That is your commitment. You have eighteen months so what is the rush? Measure when it is called for and feel the joy of success in inches lost.

Measurements

Take the following measurements. Be sure to record the date and your weight:

- Neck
- Right arm
- Left arm
- Upper chest (At under arm level)
- Chest
- Midriff (directly under the bust line)
- Waist (smallest part of the midsection)
- Hips
- Right thigh (at the largest part)
- Left thigh
- Right knee (2 inches above the top of the knee cap)
- Left knee
- Right calf (at the largest part)
- Left calf
- Other (ex. Roll 1)

Measure above the belly button and/or below the belly button. You should keep track of these measurements as these will change drastically and the waist or hip measurement will not tell you how these rolls have changed. Other areas that could be recorded that are extremely wide are areas at the top of the thighs, etc.

Avoiding Insulin Reaction Triggers

Familiar settings where you used to indulge in high carb foods can be a trigger to repeat that activity. The brain has been trained to expect certain things in that familiar place and will cause the endorphin pathway to be primed for a hit. Change things up. If you ate in front of the TV then make a point of eating somewhere else. You can drink your favorite sugar-free hot herbal tea sweetened with stevia there instead.

You will notice that the smell of baked goodies can cause you to crave carbs. This is one reason that I prefer that you determine not to make those yourself. Have the ones that will be eating it make it if that is possible, or better yet, buy them already made and keep them out of your sight.

Let us make things as easy as possible for you, especially in the beginning. As time goes on your mind and body will acquire new habits and the old insulin triggers will fade. The pleasure of living without cravings and knowing you are doing the exact best thing for your body is rather amazing.

Making Room for New

As you lose weight, take those clothes that are too big and get them out of the house. No excuses, I see you hiding under that hoodie. Give them to a thrift store where they can help someone else. You are too small for them.

There is something about keeping the old clothes that mentally tells you that it is alright to gain weight back. It is not alright. You need to be in control of that old "**Monster**" and now you have the tools to do it. Clean out that closet and get some new clothes that fit and look attractive on you. As they say, dress for success!

Eating the Rainbow

It would be so nice to give credit to whoever came up with the term "Eating the Rainbow". It is quite brilliant, such a great visual idea. I just cannot seem to find out where it originated. But at any rate, that's what you will be doing.

There's a reason that vegetables and fruits have their own bright colors. Green vegetables contain chlorophyll and powerful phytonutrients such as lutein and indoles. Yellow and orange vegetables and fruits get their pigment from alpha and beta carotenes. Blue, red and purple foods get their beautiful colors from flavonoids. We don't want to miss any of the amazing building, healing, and protective powers of these foods. This means that you need to strive to get some of each color every day.

Vegetables are full of fiber which is essential for a healthier you. It goes through the digestive track largely unaltered which means it provides little to no calories. It has a mechanical property to it, scrubbing the intestines and helping to eliminate waste. Maybe this is why it lowers the risk of certain cancers, heart disease and diabetes. Fiber helps a person feel full which can aid in weight loss.

Our goal is to get 5 to 7 vegetable servings daily. You will add fruits when you start maintenance.

The Plan

You have picked your day and are ready to start. When the day comes, you have cleared out all the foods that are not on the list. For the first week, you can eat anything on the list and as much as you want. This is so you can clear out the processed foods and all sugars from your diet. This will clear your head and there is no need to feel deprived as you can eat all you want as long as it is on the list. The first three days are the hardest. You will still experience cravings. That pleasure center of the brain is being affected It is calling for its drug of choice; sugar, refined flour, (high carb anything) and it will be hard. Expect it. You may even get sick. Headaches are common as well as some nausea.

This is a big change, the bugs you may have in your body love the acidity that processed foods and sugar gives, so you may even have die-off which can cause a Herkimer Response. This is an increase in flu-like symptoms that comes from parasites and pathogens in the blood dying off at a faster rate than their normal life cycle die off. For short it is called a Herx. Not everyone will experience this, but you may. Hold strong; this passes and you will feel better soon. Actually, the average is 3 days of some misery. And then wonders of wonders, miracles of miracles, those cravings subside and it gets so much easier.

My plan calls for abstinence, and this is what makes me different. Many other plans call for moderation and gradual reduction. This does work for some; however, in my mind, it is like pulling a band aid off slowly. It just prolongs the time when the cravings are all but gone and you can get on with things.

What a pleasure it is to be able to make wise choices about the food you will eat because you are not craving inappropriate carbs. Hunger becomes a different feeling. You will feel that you need food because you feel that decline. Not sure how else to describe it but you will know what I mean when you experience it.

Have the food choices decided in the morning. Start preparing then. If you work, get the crock pot out and have your meat choices cooking so when you get home the decisions are made. All you will need then are the vegetables, fresh and cooked.

I like to see a plate that has meat, salad, and cooked vegetables with butter or another high fat topping on it. That is a very satisfying meal. Maybe some cheese for dessert.

After the first week, remembering to weigh the same day every week, you will start counting calories. Find your BMR on the chart and reduce by about 200 calories a day. You have to eat yourself lean. If by some mysterious occurrence some addictive food gets into your mouth, spit it out before it can raise your blood sugar and cause cravings.

Continue on until you have acquired your goal weight.

This may take many months as some people are Keto resistant. Their bodies resist burning fat. Yours may also. This changes as time goes on. Some of my clients only lose ½ pound a week. It is hard for them at first but they come to realize that it does not matter, they have 18 months to achieve their weight-loss goals. A commitment is a commitment so they stay on board and great things happen. It will for you as well.

Some lose much faster. Men can commonly lose 4 pounds a week. That is hard for married couples doing the program together. Keep in mind, this is a lifestyle change for the rest of your life. Sugar addiction does not go away. I firmly believe, and this is only my opinion, that once an addict always an addict. From what I have observed, when people lose the weight they desire, they can gain all that weight back and more if they start eating their drug of choice again. That is why staying on the program is essential.

An addict out of control is misery. An addict in control, well that is an amazing life. As time goes on you stop thinking about it every moment. You may think about it every day but not all day long.

Commitment to your new slim self and accepting your new life and meal choices brings some unexpected joy. It's such a worthwhile trade off. You will find yourself finding time for things you never thought possible! When you reach your goal weight, which you will, you won't be hanging on with bloody fingernails. It will come on a day like the other days. You are in control and by the way, you look amazing because everyone tells you so!

"Taming the Monster Within" Guidelines for Weight-loss

Below are the recommended percentages of how much of each should be included in your meals:

- Protein 20-35%
- Fat 40-70%
- Carbohydrates 10-20%

Basic Guidelines

- Do not include more than 15 grams of carbohydrates in a meal
- Plan out your menu so that you eat 2 or 3 meals and 2 snacks per day
- Eat 5 to 7 vegetables each day, and vary the colors of the vegetables so you eat the rainbow
- Eat all of the day's meals and snacks within an 8-hour window
- Finish eating by 7:00 pm each day

Food choices for Weight-loss

<u>Meats</u>
- Lamb
- Red meat
- Poultry
- Seafood

- Pork
- Wild game meats

Dairy Products
- Eggs
- Cheese
- Sour cream
- Cream cheese
- Cream

Condiments
- Mayonnaise
- Mustard
- Relish (No Sugar Variety)

<u>No fruits until you reach your goal weight</u>. Lemons and limes are the exceptions.

All spices

Essential oils

Salad dressings
- Ranch
- Italian
- Any dressings without sugar

Vegetables
Try to eat a large fresh green salad daily. One serving of vegetables is one cup or the size of a small fist for green leafy vegetables, and a half cup for other vegetables.

- Artichokes
- Asparagus
- Avocado
- Bok Choy
- Broccoli
- Brussel sprouts
- Cabbage
- Carrots (limit to the shredded ones that come on salads)
- Cauliflower
- Celery
- Chives
- Cilantro
- Cocoa
- Collard Greens
- Cucumbers
- Garlic
- Green beans
- Kale
- Lettuce (all kinds)
- Mushrooms (all kinds)
- Onions (all kinds)
- Olives
- Parsley
- Parsnips
- Peppers (green, red, yellow, orange) limit to ½-1 a day
- Pickles (without sugar)
- Radishes
- Rutabaga
- Spaghetti squash
- Spinach
- Summer squash

- Swiss Chard
- Tomato (limit to one a day)
- Zucchini

Seeds and Nuts

Start to include seeds and nuts after your first week. You will be able to "feel" when a food causes an insulin spike, so after clearing your body of refined carbs, you will recognize if nuts are causing hunger. Nuts can be tricky; keep track of the carbs and calories.

- Almonds*
- Brazil nuts
- Cashews
- Chia seeds
- Coconut (can use all forms that have not been sweetened)
- Flax seeds
- Hazelnuts
- Macadamias
- Pecans
- Sesame seeds
- Sunflower seeds

*Almonds deserve a special listing as they are so low in carbs and so satisfying. Also, almond flour is a versatile replacement for refined flour in baking. Almond milk needs to be unsweetened, with or without chocolate; sweeten it with stevia.

Nut Butters
- Peanut butter (choose a variety that has no sugar added)
- Almond butter
- Sesame seed butter

Legumes (These can be eaten during your 18-month commitment when you want to eat out, chili will work for a meal at your local fast food restaurant, add the cheese and sour cream to boost the fat. Legumes are high in protein, nutrition and fiber, but they are also high in carbohydrates. When you have reached your weight-loss goals then they can be added as a regular part of your diet if you desire.)

- Beans
  - Black beans
  - Black-eyed Peas
  - Chick peas (Garbanzo beans)
  - Kidney beans
  - Lima beans
  - Navy beans
  - Northern beans
  - Pinto beans
  - Red beans
  - Soy beans
  - White beans
- Lentils
  - Yellow
  - Red
  - Green
  - Brown
  - Black

Pork rinds

Coffee or tea

Green tea has amazing benefits so this is recommended as your morning drink with MCT oil and stevia.

Fats
- Almond oil
- Butter
- Cocoa butter
- Coconut oil
- Hazelnut oil
- Lard
- MCT oil
- Olive oil
- Safflower oil
- Sesame oil
- Sunflower oil
- Walnut oil

Sweeteners
- Stevia
- Erythritol
- Xylitol

Water

Drink half your body weight each day. For example, a 120-pound person should drink a minimum of 60oz of water per day. Measure so that you can be sure you are getting this amount.

Maintenance

What a nice stage this is. You are at your goal weight. (If you have noticed I don't give guidelines for that. Everyone shakes down to a different goal weight according to what his/her bone structure is, and how they feel.) When the weight loss slows down and then really slows down, consider that you are getting close. But you are not going anywhere. We still have time before our 18 months is up. Remember you are still mine, we have 18 months together, and maintenance is part of the plan.

You are at goal weight, so you will not need to lose more weight during the remaining 18 months. Add back the calories your body can use according to your BMR. Use the same food list with the addition of low carb berries (such as strawberries and blueberries). Start with a serving of each and see how it affects your weight.

Continue to weigh yourself once a week. Did you stay the same? Or did you lose or gain weight? This tells us how you will do with adding low carb fruits. Ideally, you will stay the same as you are now at goal weight and adding a few berries should not cause you significant insulin spikes. You can feel those spikes now because you have lived for some time without that torture and you can identify them for what they are – "The Monster Within" peeking his ugly head out.

After determining how many servings of low carb fruits your body can handle and still maintain weight, it is time to figure out how much whole grain you can have without adding weight.

Start with 15 carbs of a grain once a day. Keep the calorie count within the allowed amount. After a week, weigh yourself. Did you gain any weight or did you maintain? Follow the same process that you did with the low carb fruit until you are maintaining a consistent weight from one week to the next.

Each week, experiment with different foods. Does that food cause you to crave sweets? If so, then you had an insulin reaction to that food and it is not something that should regularly be on your maintenance food list. You are going to live a life without the highs and lows of insulin spikes so keep those foods for the next step which we will talk about in a minute.

Do you love potatoes? Take heart! They are not a refined food, so try adding them to your maintenance diet in a controlled way. One medium potato has 37 carbs and 163 calories. Try having half of a medium potato at first. Make sure you add lots of butter and sour cream to slow down digestion which will limit the rise in blood sugar and any insulin reaction you may have.

Trans-fats will never be in your maintenance plan, so fried potatoes are not recommended. Oven baked French fries are pretty wonderful however. Continue on experimenting with all the foods you are interested in that do not have sugar and or white processed flours. Once you have reached goal weight continue on learning what foods can easily be on your new program. Eighteen months will come so much faster than you could have imagined. Eighteen months with absolutely no sugars and processed food, living the life of the non-addict!

The Future

Now that your eighteen-month commitment is over it is time to think about the commitment you now have for the rest of your life.

If you remember earlier, I promised that you will not be abstaining from sugar and processed foods forever. When you have completed your eighteen-month commitment and goal, you will have some decisions to make. You can have some sugar and processed foods now according to your free agency. You are free to choose the occasions when you want to eat them. You are free to choose what foods these will be.

This is how it works. Say you choose Christmas. That is always a time of year where you have lots of social gatherings with family and friends. If you do not celebrate Christmas, just think of a time that you do celebrate. On that pre-chosen day, you can decide to eat whatever you would like. It is fun to eat whatever you want to especially when treats are so prevalent.

Now it is the day after Christmas or whatever day you have chosen, and because you have completed eighteen months with abstinence you have an absolute knowledge that you can go without any more processed sugars and flours until the next time you choose. Get the treats out of your reach. Let others store them out of your sight, or throw them away. Your body can handle this type of indulgence on an occasional basis. But you are still at goal weight because you stopped the next day.

It' is awesome! You are in control, not that old "Monster Within". He'll try to be in control and tell you that you have to keep on eating that unhealthy drug of choice. But you will put him right back in his place because you know what that "Monster" is doing.

You are in control for the rest of your life because you know how to control your addiction.

With the New Year coming set some times that you will indulge again. I have a lady who loves our local bakery. She has decided that she will not look at that store and think "I can never have baked foods again." She drives by it and thinks "I will have an apple fritter in the spring." There are no thoughts of deprivation, only satisfaction that she is in control and very happy about that, and yes, she wil delay that gratification until she chooses.

Keep weighing once a week. It keeps you on track. But if time goes on and you are staying at goal weight then just go by the way your clothes fit. If you notice a difference, then stop those whole grains for a while. Only have fruit on the weekends. You will still be using the same food list with the allowances you have determined work for you. Sugar and white refined foods are never part of maintenance, only part of your chosen indulgences.

This is a wonderful life, even with the trials of mortality to which we all can relate. It is wonderful to be able to be engaged in life without the burden of addiction. It is like taking off a heavy, hot itchy dark coat that is not comfortable in any way. You have unbuttoned it and you step away. You look back at it and realize how that controlled your life and there was nothing good about it. You feel light and unburdened.

You are excited for new challenges and ready to go forward with the new adventures of life, ready to be there for your loved ones and all those who may need your help. Ready to be an example because that is how you live your life. Be excited about new technologies, scientific advancements, the arts, music, and literature. Who knows? Your new life style may possibly give you more days to enjoy on this earth.

Living with our addictions under control gives us more time for other things. You might write a book about your passion! You will not need to be afraid of the "**Monster Within**" ever again.

You should be so proud of yourself! I know I am!

In Retrospect

Before beginning "The Plan", the old you wakes up, looks in the mirror, and thinks, "I have to do something about this! I know! I won't eat hardly anything today and I will exercise. But which exercise? And when will I have time? Well, it doesn't matter. I have to exercise off those cookies I made yesterday so this is more important than anything else."

With the day centered around undoing your previous indulgence, you now have to play catch up because going to the gym took all morning. However, the exercise paid off because now you are feeling better about things. Lunch is decidedly low carb. Yep, things are better. Nevertheless, anxiety starts to creep in and turns into a primitive type of fear as you start to consider the afternoon without sugar. The kids get off the bus around four, and you want to be a great Mom or Dad, so you better make a treat. The kids love those chocolate chip cookies. You'll just have to make those.

While making the cookies, you have to try the batter. It is so amazing, you have to have a least one cookie. But you can't eat a cookie without milk. The kids come home, awe and ooh over them, and have one or two as they go off to play. You stay there, cleaning up the mess, and eat way past the point of feeling full. Pretty soon you reach that degree of self-loathing and reproach which always follows in these situations. "Okay," you say to yourself, "it's all right. I will exercise even more tomorrow." This cycle repeats itself over and over creating a deeper sense of disappointment.

Or perhaps you are on the go working. You didn't pack a lunch, which you usually don't. That takes too much time. Which fast food restaurant will you choose today? It is not your fault the number 7 is loaded with trans-fats, high carbs, and calories. It is a full meal deal, right?

You will do something about your increasing waistline and further decline towards diabetes and heart disease tomorrow.

After Eighteen Months

But now you've made it this far in "The Plan". The new you wakes up, looks in the mirror, and thinks, "I look fine. No really, I look just fine! What should I do today? Whom shall I show love and attention to? Whom shall I serve? What goals can I work on?"

This is a wonderful way to start the day! You have your morning to get things done, and since you are fresh from a great night of sleep, you get on top of the challenges of the day. Exercise is easier to fit into your day, because you don't feel the need to do an extreme workout.

You know that sugar is not an option, so when four o'clock rolls around and the kids are off the bus, they come home to a snack of celery with old fashioned peanut butter (that has no sugar added) and maybe some raisins to make it look like ants on a log. You eat the celery and peanut butter, decide not to put on the raisins, and feel completely satisfied with an appropriate serving. The kids are happy and think Mom (or Dad) is great.

Or you might be at work where you wave the donut cart on, and the guy selling them just smiles. He is used to you. Driving by fast food chains is quieter now; they are not calling your name. There are no thoughts of disappointment in yourself or promises to make things better by over exercising. It is not necessary. You already did the hard work by making correct decisions which were possible because you were not struggling from insulin reactions and sugar addiction cravings.

Maintenance is a lifestyle. You will not bring in the misery of high carb refined foods which will most definitely awaken food cravings. The first eighteen months of commitment should be a prelude to a life of commitment. This new life is your new norm.

Some On-going Thoughts

There are some things that I want to talk with you about before our conversation ends.

An addiction can only be managed through abstinence. Sugar addiction becomes possible to overcome when the insulin production and consequently insulin spikes are controlled. The insulin spike is the culprit that causes major food cravings. It follows that to control insulin spikes you will be eating a low carb diet. Eating low carb is healthy and satisfying and will give a person the weight loss he/she desires. Low carb eating is maintainable in the fashion I have outlined, giving people the free agency to choose when and where they would like to indulge in high carb foods with a return to healthy eating immediately after. It is abstinence with a twist!

Another thing is that you will need to protect your new life and body. You should not be casual about this, as you have gone through a lot to get your body and health where you want it. It is not your responsibility to eat other people's treats. People can be food pushers and not even realize it. Or maybe they do- misery loves company. Whatever the situation may be, if it is not a choice you have previously made to indulge that day, pleasantly decline. Their happiness is not your responsibility.

Your happiness and success are your responsibility. You look great. You feel great. Let's keep it that way.

Take care of any weight gain right away. It is easy to get back by implementing your first week again. Eat all you want of the appropriate foods which are filling and satisfying. The second week will be continuing on with choosing from the list of food that is unprocessed, unrefined, real food. You have experience in how much food your body can utilize, and getting your calories to an appropriate amount is like going back home. You feel comfortable there. When your appetite spikes, it is because your insulin spikes and that happens when you eat high carb food. Get that "Monster Within" back into his box and your appetite gets right back into your control.

Keep on preparing and cooking delicious food, this is a key to ongoing success.

I think you are wonderful!
BE HAPPY. You deserve it!

References

1.Keith Kantor, PDH, a nutritionist was quoted in the Huffington Post 6/9/2014

2. Food in History, Reay Tannahill, 1988, Crown Publishers, Inc. New York P.319

3. How Sugar is made-the History SKIL May 15th, 2016

4. JenniferRegan http://BambooCorefitness/ article/December10,2014

5. Salt, Sugar, Fat by Micheal Moss, Random House, New York, copyright 2013

6.Avena NM, Rada P, Hoebel BG. Evidence for sugar addiction: behavioral and neurochemical effects of intermittent, excessive sugar intake. Neurosci Biobehav Rev. 2008;32(1):20-39. Epub 2007 May 18.

7. Mark Hyman M.D./ drhyman.com/ blog/2013/06/27/5-clues-you-are-addicted-to-sugar/

8. THIQ = Tetrahydroisoquinoline http://callais.net/FS_EDU_THIQ.html

9. The Neurobiology of Drug Addiction/The ActionofHeroin(Morphine)/Definition/dependence/www.drugab

use.gov/publications/teaching-packets/neurobiology-drug-addiction/

10. Post Register/Sept/13/2016 Exposing Sugar/front page/ Associated Press/

11. Gerald F.M. Russell, 1979 /Bulimia Nervosa/ written by Dr. Viveanand, Published on Nov. 27, 2014

12. A History of Eating Disorders by Emily Deans M.D. /posted Dec. 11, 2011/ image credit (wikipedia)

13. Clinical Diabetes/ Vol. 18 NO. 2 Spring 2000/ Barbara A. Ramlo-Halsted, MD and Steven V. Edelman, MD

14. Greene JA, Prescribing by numbers. Drugs and the definition of disease. John Hopkins University Press, 2007

15. Dietary Assessment of Major Trends in US Food Consumption, 1970-2005. Hodan Farah Wells and Jean C. Buzby/ www.ers.usda.gov

16. Statistics on Weight Descrimination: A Waste of Talent, The Council on Size and Weight Descrinimation, retrieved July 18th, 2011/www.cswd.org/index.html

17. FoodAddictsAnonymous http://www.foodaddictsanonymous.org/abstinence

18. Mercola/DrRonRosedale,M.D./articles.mercola.com/sites/articles/archive/2001/07/14insulin-part-one.aspx

19. Nancy Appleton P.H.D. http://home.earthlink.net/-loveguru/NOSUGAR.htm 2/21/2013

20.ChicagoTribune.com/lifestyles/health/sc-humans-longevity-limit-health-1019-20161006-story,html

21. Shredded Wheat Dishes/Copyright 1910/ The Shredded Wheat Company/Niagara Falls, N.Y.

22. The Perricone Weight Loss Diet/ Nicholas Perricone, M.D./ Ballantine Books/New York/2005/p.102/

23.TheWashingtonPost/RobertoA.Ferdman/https://www.washingtonpost.com/news/wonk/wp/2015/02/05/where-people-around-the-world-eat-the-most-sugar

24.The Candida Diet, last updated january 15, 2017 by Lisa Richards, https://www.thecandidadiet.com/acetaldehyde-and-candida/

25. 5 Reasons Cancer and Sugar are Best Friends/article/

2014 - 03 – 09 http://beatcancer.org/blog-posts/5-reasons-cancer-and-sugar-are-best-friends/

26. Gatenby RA. Potential role of FDG-PET imaging in understanding tumor-host interaction. J Nucl Med 1995 May;36(5):893-9.

27 NutritionRole of sugars in human neutrophilic phagocytosis1,2Albert Sanchez, J. L. Reeser, H. S. Lau, P. Y. Yahiku, R. E. Willard, P. J. McMillan,S. Y. Cho27.The American Journal of Clinical, A. R. Magie, and U. D. Register http://ajcn.nutrition.org/content/26/11/1180.abstractCopyright © 1973 by The American Society for Clinical Nutrition, Inc

28. The History of Food Fortification in the United States: Its Relevance for Current Fortification Efforts in Developing

Countries Author(s): David Bishai and Ritu Nalubola Source: Economic Development and Cultural Change, Vol. 51, No. 1 (October 2002), pp. 37-53 Published by: The University of Chicago Press Stable URL: http://www.jstor.org/stable/10.1086/34536

29. 2 de Munter JS, Hu FB, Spiegelman D, Franz M, van Dam RM. Whole grain, bran, and germ intake and risk of type 2 diabetes: a prospective cohort study and systematic review. PLoS Med

30. Health News, May 27, 2011/12:42pm/. www.reuters.com/article/us-msg-linked-weight-gain-idUSTRE74Q5SJ20110527/ Adam Marcus **"MSG linked to weight gain"**

31. Br J Clin Pharmacol. 2002 Jun; 53(6): 641643.doi: 10.1046/j.13652125.2002.01596.x PMCID: PMC1874333/Effects of oral monosodium (L)-glutamate on insulin secretion and glucose tolerance in healthy volunteers
Hugues Chevassus,[1] Eric Renard,[2] Gyslaine Bertrand,[3] Isabelle Mourand,[1] Raymond Puech,[3] Nathalie Molinier,[1] Joël Bockaert,[3] Pierre Petit,[1] and Jacques Bringer[2]

32. Monosodium Glutamate (MSG) literally stimulates neurons to death ... Dr. Russell Blaylock, M.D, Board certifiedneurosurgeonhttps://www.pinterest.com/pin/109986415869542320/

33. http://www.msgexposed .com/studies-show-msg-fed-mice-became-gross

34. Richard I. Horowitz, MD, Why Can't I get Better? St Martin's press, New York, 2013, p.235

35. Harvard Health Blog » Eating too much added sugar increases the risk of dying with heart disease - Harvard Health Blog, posted february 06, 2014, 2:04 pm , updated november 30, 2016, 3:29 pm
Julie Corliss, Executive Editor, Harvard Heart Letter

36.*NeuroImage*
Volume 55, Issue 1, 1 March 2011, Pages 420-433/https://www.ncbi.nlm.nih.gov/pmc/articles/PMC3031763/

37. Kubo K, Iinuma M, Chen H. Mastication as a Stress-Coping Behavior. *BioMed Research International.* 2015: 1-11.

38. Dr Joseph Mercola, "Fat for Fuel" Hayhouse, Inc. copyright 2017

39. Nature. 2014 Oct 9;514(7521):181-6. doi: 10.1038/nature13793. Epub 2014 Sep 17.Artificial sweeteners induce glucose intolerance by altering the gut microbiota. carrying nutrients and oxygen to your cell

40.Published online 2014 May 14. doi: 10.1002/ijc.28809Ketone supplementation decreases tumor cell viability and prolongs survival of micewithmetastaticcancer/www.ncbi.nlm.nih.gov/pmc/articles/PMC4235292/AM Poff,1 C Ari,1 P Arnold,2 TN Seyfried,3 and DP D'Agostino1

41.https://www.ncbi.nlm.nih.gov/pubmed/15640462 Am J Clin Nutr. 2005 Jan;81(1):69-73.Alternate-day fasting in nonobese subjects: effects on body weight, body composition, and energy metabolism.Heilbronn LK1, Smith SR, Martin CK, Anton SD, Ravussin E.

42. Translational Research, vol 164, Issue 4, October 2014,Pages 302-311 In-Depth Review: Excess Adiposity and Disease, Intermittent fasting vs daily calorie restriction for type 2 diabetes prevention: a review of human findings

43.www.ncbi.nlm.nih.gov/pmc/articles/PMC329619/

doi: 10.1172/JCI113450Fasting enhances growth hormone secretion and amplifies the complex rhythms of growth hormone secretion in man.

K Y Ho, J D Veldhuis, M L Johnson, R Furlanetto, W S Evans, K G Alberti, and M O Thorner

44.www.ncbi.nlm.nih.gov/pmc/articles/PMC3106288/Autophagy . 2010 Aug 16; 6(6): 702–710. Published online 2010 Aug 14. doi: 10.4161/auto.6.6.12376Short-term fasting induces profound neuronal autophagy

Mehrdad Alirezaei,#1 Christopher C. Kemball,#1 Claudia T. Flynn,1 Malcolm R. Wood,2 J. Lindsay Whitton, 1 and William B. Kiosses2

45.Am J Physiol. 1990 Jan;258(1 Pt 2):R87-93.Enhanced thermogenic response to epinephrine after 48-h starvation inhumans.Mansell PI1, Fellows IW, Macdonald IA.

46. BioMed Research International, Volume 2014 (2014), Article ID 761264, 19 pages http://dx.doi.org/10.1155/2014/761264Review ArticleOxidative Stress, Prooxidants, and Antioxidants: The Interplay

47.Free Radic Biol Med. 2007 Mar 1;42(5):665-74. Epub 2006 Dec 14.

Alternate day calorie restriction improves clinical findings and reduces markers of oxidative stress and inflammation in overweight adults with moderate asthma.Johnson JB1, Summer W, Cutler RG, Martin B, Hyun DH, Dixit VD, Pearson M, Nassar M, Telljohann R, Maudsley S, Carlson O, John S, Laub DR, Mattson MP. /www.ncbi.nlm.nih.gov/pubmed/17291990/

48.www.ncbi.nlm.nih.gov/pubmed/19793855Am J Clin Nutr. 2009 Nov;90(5):1138-43. doi: 10.3945/ajcn.2009.28380. Epub 2009 Sep 30.Short-term modified alternate-day fasting: a novel dietary strategy for weight loss and cardioprotection in obese adults.Varady KA1, Bhutani S, Church EC, Klempel MC.

49. Neurobiol Dis. 2007 pr:26 (1):212-20. Epub 2007 Jan 13. Intermittent fasting and caloric restriction ameliorate age-related behavioral deficits in the triple-transgenic mouse model of Alzheimer's'disease. www.ncbi.nlm.nih.gov/pubmed/17306982

50. First published March 29, 2017, doi: 10.3945/ajcn.116.142158Am J Clin Nutr May 2017 vol. 105 no. 5 1239-1247 A systematic review and meta-analysis of randomized controlled trials of the effect of konjac glucomannan, a viscous soluble fiber, on LDL cholesterol and the new lipid targets non-HDL cholesterol and apolipoprotein B1,2

51. Tokai J Exp Clin Med. 1990 Nov;15(6):417-23.Effects of berberine, a plant alkaloid, on the growth of anaerobic protozoa in axenic culture

52. East Afr Med J. 1997 May;74(5):283-4.Treatment of chloroquine-resistant malaria using pyrimethamine in combination with berberine, tetracycline or cotrimoxazole.

53.CandidaYeastProtectionProgram/JimEnglish/nutritionreview.

org/2013/04/candida/yeast-protection-program-part2/

54. Eur J Pharmacol. 2008 Jul 28;589(1-3):163-72. doi:
10.1016/j.ejphar.2008.05.043. Epub 2008 Jun 3.

On the mechanism of antidepressant-like action of berberine
chloride.

55. Eur J Pharmacol. 2013 Jan 5;698(1-3):259-66. doi:
10.1016/j.ejphar.2012.10.020. Epub 2012 Oct 23.Hippocampal
synaptic plasticity restoration and anti-apoptotic effect underlie
berberine improvement of learning and memory in
streptozotocin-diabetic rats.

56. J Infect Dis. 2011 Jun 1;203(11):1602-12.
doi:10.1093/infdis/jir147.Berberine ameliorates intestinal
epithelial tight-junction damage and down-regulates myosin light
chain kinase pathways in a mouse model of endotoxinemia.

57. Sci Rep. 2016 Mar 3;6:22612. doi: 10.1038/srep22612.
Berberine Ameliorates Hepatic Steatosis and Suppresses Liver
and Adipose Tissue Inflammation in Mice with Diet-induced
Obesity.

58. Biochem Pharmacol. 2012 Nov 15;84(10):1260-7. doi:
10.1016/j.bcp.2012.07.018. Epub 2012 Jul 25.Berberine: new
perspectives for old remedies

59. Biochem Biophys Res Commun. 2007 Nov 3;362(4):853-7.
Epub 2007 Aug 27.Berberine-induced LDLR up-regulation
involves JNK pathway.

60. Effects of berberine on angiotensin-converting enzyme and
NO/cGMP system in vessels Department of Herbal Resources,

Professional Graduate School of Oriental Medicine and Medicinal Resources Research Center (MRRC), Wonkwang University, Iksan, Chonbuk, 570-749, Republic of KoreaReceived 1 January 2002, Accepted 1 February 2002, Available online 3 April 2003

61. Mol Med Rep. 2013 Feb;7(2):461-5. doi: 10.3892/mmr.2012.1236. Epub 2012 Dec 14.Berberine attenuated monocyte adhesion to endothelial cells induced by oxidized low density lipoprotein via inhibition of adhesion molecule expression.

Huang Z1, Cai X, Li S, Zhou H, Chu M, Shan P, Huang W.

62. Biochem Biophys Res Commun. 2007 Jan 12;352(2):498-502. Epub 2006 Nov 15.Berberine alters the processing of Alzheimer's amyloid precursor protein to decrease Abeta secretion.

63. Exp Biol Med (Maywood). 2011 Jul;236(7):859-66. doi: 10.1258/ebm.2011.010366. Epub 2011 Jun 15. Effects of berberine on human rheumatoid arthritis fibroblast-like synoviocytes.

64. Phytother Res. 2011 Jun;25(6):878-85. doi: 10.1002/ptr.3359. Epub 2010 Nov 24.Protective effects of berberine in an experimental rat osteoarthritis model.Hu PF1, Chen WP, Tang JL, Bao JP, Wu LD.

65. Clin Exp Pharmacol Physiol. 2008 Mar;35(3):303-9. Epub 2007 Oct 30.Protection by and anti-oxidant mechanism of berberine against rat liver fibrosis induced by multiple hepatotoxic facyors

66. Eur J Pharmacol. 2011 Jan 25;651(1-3):187-96. doi: 10.1016/j.ejphar.2010.10.030. Epub 2010 Oct 20. Evidence for the complementary and synergistic effects of the three-alkaloid combination regimen containing berberine, hypaconitine and skimmianine on the ulcerative colitis rats

67. Inflammation. 2012 Jun;35(3):841-9. doi: 10.1007/s10753-011-9385-6.Berberine ameliorates pro-inflammatory cytokine-induced endoplasmic reticulum stress in human intestinal epithelial cells in vitro

68.IntImmunopharmacol.2011Nov;11(11):1706-14. doi: 10.1016/j.intimp.2011.06.002. Epub 2011 Jun 16.Inhibition of H1N1 influenza A virus growth and induction of inflammatory mediators by the isoquinoline alkaloid berberine and extracts of goldenseal (Hydrastis canadensis).Cecil CE1, Davis JM, Cech NB, Laster SM.

69. Mol Biol Rep. 2013 Jun;40(6):3913-23. doi: 10.1007/s11033-012-2468-0. Epub 2012 Dec 25 Berberine ameliorates renal injury by regulating G proteins-AC- cAMP signaling in diabetic rats with nephropathy.Tang LQ1, Wang FL, Zhu LN, Lv F, Liu S, Zhang ST.

70. Biochim Biophys Acta. Author manuscript; available in PMC 2012 Jun 4.Published in final edited form as:Biochim Biophys Acta. 2012 Feb; 1822(2): 185–195.Published online 2011 Oct 17. doi: 10.1016/j.bbadis.2011.10.008, Berberine protects against high fat diet-induced dysfunction in muscle mitochondria by inducing SIRT1-dependent mitochondrial biogenesis, Ana P. Gomes,a,b Filipe V. Duarte,a Patricia Nunes,a Basil P. Hubbard,b João S. Teodoro,a Ana T. Varela,a John G.

71. Dr Joseph Mercola, "Fat for Fuel" page 251, Hayhouse, Inc. copyright 2017

72. Kolanowski J, deGasparo M, Desmecht P, Crabbe J (1972) Further evaluation of the role of insulin in sodium retention associated with carbohydrate administration after a fast in the obese. Eur J Clin Invest 2: 439–444

73. Reverse Osmosis Water- A Poor Product, by Dr. Lawrence Wilson Copyright 2013, L.D. Wilson Consultants, Inc.

www.ingramcontent.com/pod-product-compliance
Lightning Source LLC
Chambersburg PA
CBHW071401280526
45787CB00001B/403